DYING
IN THE LAND
OF
PLENTY

DYING
IN THE LAND
OF
PLENTY

UNVEILING THE SHROUD OF DISEASE

by
Brenda O. Brown

MARPE´ PUBLISHING . **New York**

ISBN: 0-9716724-0-7

Library of Congress Control Number: 2002090795

First Printing: September 2002

Cover Design: Edward Hettig and Sandi Sheldon
Editors: Tina Finneyfrock, and Barbara Hayes
Page Layout: THE WRITING BRANCH - Sylvia McNitt
Photographer: PICTURES WITH PRIDE - Tom Szewczyk

Printed and bound in the United States of America

DISCLAIMER

ATTENTION: ORGANIZATIONS, HEALING CENTERS, AND SCHOOLS OF SPIRITUAL DEVELOPEMENT AND HEALTHY LIFESTYLES - Quantity discounts are available on bulk purchases of this book for educational purposes and fund raising. Special books or book excerpts can also be created to fit specific needs. For information please contact: Marpe´ Solutions, 523 Granville Hill Road, Sherburne, NY 13460 - Attn: Brenda O. Brown

To my precious son W. Logan,
who was the driving force behind
my healing.   May the trials we have
endured and the triumphs we have soared to,
forever bind us in
God's love and mercy.

Mom

ACKNOWLEDGMENTS

I submit a reverent utterance of praise and thanksgiving to my heavenly Father who allowed me to bear this cross, strengthening my faith and desire to help others.

My sincere gratitude and admiration to Dr. Kalpana Patel, who cares enough for mankind that she dedicates her life to continued research and study in the cause and prevention of disease and suffering. A special thanks to Debbie Napieracz, her nurse, for the passion and expertise with which she performs her duties.

My heartfelt appreciation to the various physicians and nurses who served behind the scenes during my recovery, most notably, Dr. Richard Ucci, Dr. Chester Clark, and Kevin Steckline, RPA.

I forever remain indebted to my special friend, Joe Salem, for his part in the seemingly endless search to locate a doctor that was able to properly diagnose my illness. Without him, my story would have had a very different conclusion.

My most humble thanks to my church family for their never ceasing prayers and encouragement through my illness.

"And the prayer of faith shall save the sick, and the Lord shall raise him up, and if he have committed sins, they shall be forgiven him. Confess your faults one to another, and pray one for another, that ye may be healed. The effectual fervent prayer of a righteous man availeth much."

- *James 5: 15 and 16*

With loving appreciation to my family and friends, who kept an ever-present vigil on my progress. These folks ignored their own needs to help me through my daily struggles.

To all of you.....your love, care, and compassion will be forever etched upon my heart.

Brenda O. Brown

FOREWORD

This book offers hope to many and provides information on how patients can begin to improve their own health through avoidance of pollutants in the air, food, water, and proper nutrition. Health is something to be greatly desired by the ill, who need to be gently guided in learning to help themselves. Brenda Brown has shown easy to follow steps, recognizing and overcoming common problems.

The Chinese have a saying- "Disease enters through the mouth." This author has also discussed food as a contributing factor in the development of disease, which often was thought to be an unorthodox alternative. She has also emphasized the substance behind well-known adages such as- "Your body doesn't lie," and "You are what you eat, breathe and drink."

The most successful treatment that we have at the Environmental Health Center in Buffalo, for environmentally ill patients, is the reduction of the total body pollutant load. This book is a map for guiding anyone traveling the road from ill health to optimal health.

Kalpana D. Patel, M.D.
Director of Allergy & Environmental
Health Center of Western New York
President of American Board of Environmental Medicine

PREFACE

A vast amount of misinformation is being distributed concerning diet, health, sickness, disease, food, nutrition, cancer, drugs, and weight-loss. The list seems endless. This book was written in an effort to educate the reader in lifestyle changes and natural alternatives to health care. This book is not meant to be an exhaustive desk reference, but a common sense approach to achieving renewed health. I am confident this vital information will instill a burning desire in you to continue fighting until an answer is found for your illness and you embark upon your road to recovery. Do not give up!

The information and opinions provided must not be used in place of a physician or qualified health care practitioner. It is designed for use in conjunction with the services provided by physicians practicing, or receptive to, natural medicine. I strongly urge you to develop a good relationship with a physician knowledgeable in the art and science of natural and preventive medicine. You must take control of your own health, choosing lifestyles and methods of treatment that will ensure a long, healthy life. Before you read or research further, realize that it is you and only you that can take the first step, in improving your health and your family's health.

People are very peculiar creatures. We all want to be healthy, but refuse to work at our good health. Americans take more time and energy to research the type of car or home they wish to purchase, than they do in maintaining their health. The United States spends more money worldwide in healthcare costs for treatment than any other country. It is also the lowest rated in forms of preventative care and actual positive results obtained from "high technology." Sometimes it is the simplest of measures that can create the most dramatic effects. Even though the scientific community has proven cigarette smoking and excessive drinking of alcohol can cause disease and death, we still do it. We continue until a shocking diagnosis causes us to quit, or a loved one is diagnosed with cirrhosis of the liver or lung cancer. Suddenly, the willpower to stop the habit exhibits itself. Our tendency to overindulge in anything usually continues until symptoms rear their ugly heads, often too late to correct the problem.

Temperance is an important key to a healthy lifestyle as well as avoidance, whenever possible, of known toxins to our body. Excessive smoking, drinking, eating, etc., can and does have a negative impact on the body. Why be reactive when being proactive can lead to a healthy body and improved quality of life? Instead of waiting for our bodies to reject our ways of life, we need to become proactive and pursue a body that portrays a picture of health.

We can't continuously work and live in the industrial pollution of heavy metals and chemicals without them being absorbed or inhaled into our bodies. How much can our bodies take prior to becoming so toxic and sick, that we can no longer get out of bed in the morning?

How much stress from the corporate world and the vision of reaching the top at any cost, can our bodies tolerate? How many fourteen-hour days will we put in before realizing our children have grown and left home? Then, we may be left to live the remainder of our days alone with a dreaded illness. When will we wake up to the many warning signals within our bodies that are pointing us toward a life of destruction?

In the wake of many incurable diseases each of us is responsible for our own health and well being. It is time to take the heat off the physicians and respect them for whom and what they are. Let us not get to the point where we have abused our bodies so badly that we need to seek surgeons to do transplants, clean out our arteries, perform bypass surgeries and treat our symptoms with poisonous drugs. Prevention is the key and it is our responsibility, not that of our doctor. Let's encourage our physicians to become more involved with our healing process, allowing them to pass the knowledge they gain with each illness to the next patient.

¤¤¤

As Dr. Michael Murray and Dr. Joseph Pizzorno alluded to in the Encyclopedia of Natural Medicine and to which I have added (see Bibliography).

Instead of

- Looking at the body as a machine, treat the whole patient.

- Separating the body and mind, realize they are intricately interconnected.

- Emphasizing the elimination of disease, strive to achieve good health.

- Treating the symptoms, treat the underlying illness.

- Specializing, take an integrated approach.

- Using high technology, focus on diet, lifestyle changes and preventative measures.

- Making the physician emotionally neutral, include them in the caring and empathy of the patient, which is critical to total healing.

- Making the physician the all-knowing authority, employ them in a partnership in the healing process.

- Placing the physician in control of the patient's health decisions, place the patient in charge of health care choice.

- Trying to do it all on our own, ask God to guide and direct us in all that we do. He has promised to give wisdom to those that ask.

~

Let's take responsibility for our well being and good health. Time is running out! Today is the first day of being proactive toward your own well-being.

Today is the day!

~

"The doctor of the future will give no medicine but will interest his patients in the care of the human frame, in diet, and in the course and prevention of disease."

- Thomas A. Edison

"Every calling is great when greatly pursued."
- Oliver Wendell Holmes Jr.

Table of Contents

INTRODUCTION

The Untold Story

As a new dawn broke upon Granville Hill, I opened my eyes to the realization that I had survived another night, another long, sleepless and agonizing night, filled with pain and gut wrenching nausea.

As I slowly focused my eyes on the clock of my bedroom wall, I mindlessly watched as seconds painstakingly ticked by. The background of the clock pictured a flock of geese soaring gracefully above a familiar body of water. Grouped together as one, they glided effortlessly through the lower heavens. A realization of loneliness and abandonment suddenly swept over me.

"Oh God where are you?" I thought. "Why have you allowed this to happen to me? When will it end?" As the same questions I had asked every day for the last two years filled my mind, I glanced at the "Footprints" picture hanging on the wall near my bed.

If God was truly carrying me through this death-defying ordeal, as the infamous poem quoted, then why didn't I feel his presence? Why didn't he give me a sign that this agony would soon end? The silence was deafening.

Lying motionless, I pondered on the full and active life I had once known. Little by little, symptom by symptom, my life was being snuffed out. It seemed like ages since I had taken disability and left my stressful career in telecommunications. My home had become my prison. I no longer ran with my little four-year-old son or laughed with my friends.

I reminisced about the wonderful and joyous times I had experienced with my son and what a miracle he was to me. I thought of the many years I battled infertility, recalling the extensive testing and procedures I had endured hoping for a child. Seventeen years later, finally giving up the struggle, I did at last conceive. I had been blessed with a beautiful baby boy. As the flashing thought of death and abandoning my child passed through my mind, I cried out to God for another miracle. "Please God, I don't want to go, not now," was my plea. Again the cries were drowned in silence.

After drenching my pillowcase in tears for what seemed an eternity, I decided it was time to quit feeling self pity and get out of bed. As I pulled myself up and out of bed, supporting myself by items of furniture along the way, I settled into my rocking chair in the next room. Reaching for the phone book, I secretly hoped today, would be the day, I found a doctor that could diagnose my illness.

Attempts at a diagnosis had proven futile in the past, leaving me in a downward spiral. I had been referred to many physicians who prescribed various drugs and procedures in an effort to remedy my illness. Needless and life altering surgeries, which included the removal of my gallbladder, partial removal of my stomach and a radical hysterectomy had left me scarred both physically and emotionally.

In an effort to control the pain of my despair, one doctor prescribed Prozac. Rejecting the suggested drug, I came to the realization that the standard medical community believed this illness was emotional. Sobbing, I lashed out, "Of course it's emotional, I am very sick, in pain from head to toe and no human being can tell me what is wrong." That day, much to the displeasure of the medical staff, I discharged myself from the hospital, vowing never to return. I pledged at that moment, that if I were to die, it would be at home with dignity and peace, in the presence of my family. My brother honored my request and drove me home.

Once again, I turned my focus to the business at hand finding two additional doctors specializing in gastrointestinal disorders. Although the symptoms I displayed left no parts of my body unaffected, I felt these doctors might offer some hope. The doctor who had arranged for the last two major surgeries, openly shared with me his perplexity of my illness and the fact that my symptoms had not responded to the surgeries. At the advice of close friends and due to the desperate state of health I was in, I also contacted a facility specializing in alternative and natural healing methods. Although unfamiliar with alternative medicine, I felt I had nothing to lose. After placing several hopeful calls, I decided to return to bed to await a call.

As I slowly scuffed by the full-length mirror hanging on my bedroom door, I turned in disgust as I viewed my frail, lifeless body. In the last year I had lost over fifty pounds, bottoming out at eighty-nine pounds. Most of my hair had fallen out and my skin was sallow in color. I resembled a prisoner of war dwelling in a concentration camp. It was difficult to imagine that a few years earlier I had been an aerobics instructor.

The phone finally rang and my Aunt Bernice, who had come to live and care for me, quickly brought the phone to my bedside. One of the physicians practicing at a well-known hospital in New York returned my call, scheduling me for an appointment the following month. As I graciously accepted the appointment, a dubious thought fleeted through my mind, as I wondered if I would even be alive by then. Unspoken words and guarded expressions by family and friends didn't conceal the certainty of my spiraling demise.

Approximately one week later, Joe, a friend and former co-worker, called to inquire how I was doing. Informed that my health was declining further and perplexed that no doctor was able to diagnose the illness, he decided to do some research on his own. Later that same week, Joe phoned to say that after many phone calls, conversations and referrals he had located a doctor specializing in environmental medicine in Buffalo, New York. He contacted the doctor and explained the severity of the circumstances. An appointment was scheduled immediately.

Three days later, I felt the ever so familiar ker-plunck, ker-plunck sound of the expansion joints in the pavement on the interstate. I would have found the constant and repetitious sound annoying in times past; however, now it carried me into an almost hypnotic state, as I lay motionless in the back seat of the van. Toni and Dick, close friends from my church, had once again so generously offered to make another hopeful trip with me. Not wishing to disturb me, they conversed quietly as they drove. Drifting in and out, I silently prayed that this visit would be the one that could give me back the life I once had known.

Upon arriving at the doctor's office, Toni answered most of the routine questions, as I was incoherent much of the time. My thought process was confused and disoriented. However, I distinctly remember a particular question that infuriated me. The doctor asked, "What are your hobbies?" The adrenaline rushed through me as I thought of the absurdity of this question. I was lying on my deathbed and she wanted to know what I did for fun!

I mumbled that before becoming ill, I involved myself in the restoration of an old Victorian-style home. Little did I realize, the answer to that question would be the key in diagnosing my illness and the beginning of a very long recovery process.

A multitude of questions, a complete physical, a series of blood tests, and a 24-hour urine collection ensued. The doctor requested that I return in three days for two days of allergy testing, which would continue for two days, every week, for one month. My body was battered, my spirit almost broken. No longer could I eat a morsel of food or drink water without experiencing excruciating pain.

After all testing and evaluations, I was diagnosed as having heavy metal and chemical poisoning. Mercury and lead were at severely toxic levels and many other metals were found to be moderately toxic. High levels of benzene, xylene, as well as other chemicals were embedded within the tissues of my body. Multiple mineral and vitamin deficiencies due to my inability to eat and absorb food, as well as the damage done to my intestinal tract by the toxins, had left me severely malnourished.

My doctor explained the critical and demanding protocol I would need to follow. It was so overwhelming that I wondered if I had the strength and willpower to persist. The metals and chemicals, failed treatments, x-rays, surgeries, and drugs had taken their toll. I had an extremely toxic body and steps needed to be taken immediately to reverse this condition to save my life.

My body was so broken, it had become allergic to most every substance in the environment. At the end of the first month of treatment, I was taking three injections per day of twenty-two different antigens. The antigens consisted of molds, pollens, dust, grasses, trees, foods, and chemicals.

Looking back, I vividly remember all the weekly nutritional IV's and chelation therapy sessions I sat through. I endured over 600 saunas to sweat out the chemicals and bounced thousands of times on a mini trampoline that served as an internal chelator. I have consumed hundreds of supplements to help detoxify and rebuild my immune system. My home experienced a complete makeover, resulting in a much healthier place to dwell. I researched what foods heal and what foods harm and what drinking lots of pure water and breathing clean air could do for my health. I realized stress and lack of sleep are the ultimate killers. A dollar value can never be attached to the wealth of knowledge I gained through my recovery process.

Remarkably, in January 2000, I returned to my career in telecommunications. I am now once again the mother that God intended me to be, laughing and playing with my son, who is now 11 years old.

Tonight, as I sit relaxing in the same rocking chair where I spent many long and lonely hours, I am very aware that God was indeed carrying me through all those horrendous times. I shudder to think what the outcome may have been if he had not been at my side. God granted me a second miracle, not the instantaneous miracle where a blind person was made to see, or a lame person made able to walk, but a miracle of trust, belief, persistence, patience, discipline, love and ultimate healing. I no longer even resemble that once sick and dying person. My heart has changed as well; consequently, my life has changed.

Much of my time is now spent writing and counseling others in the cause and prevention of disease, as well as teaching effective steps that can be taken to heal a broken and toxic body. I was granted a second chance at life, as well as an education by experience, and the opportunity and passion to share this knowledge with others. As I bound out of bed each morning, I secretly wonder how many lives I will reach today.

Faith, determination, education and discipline can turn a seemingly hopeless situation into an opportunity to not only better our own lives but also the lives of others. I am so thankful to God, my doctor and the many friends and family members that reached out to me in my hour of need.

God's timing is perfect. He is in the process of designing a patchwork quilt of my life and continues to weave it daily. My goal is now to help others understand the pattern he is weaving within the patchwork quilt of their lives.

My hope is that as you read this book, the knowledge passed on to you will be life changing for you, as well as those lives touching yours.

May you grow in knowledge and understanding as you search for answers, realizing healthy lifestyle changes will bring renewed hope and the good health you were meant to have.

~

FOOTPRINTS IN THE SAND

One night a man had a dream. He dreamed he was walking along the beach with the Lord. Across the sky flashed scenes from his life. For each scene, he noticed two sets of foot prints in the sand: One belonging to him, and the other to the Lord.

When the last scene of his life flashed before him, he looked back at the footprints in the sand. He noticed that many times along the path of his life there was only one set of footprints. He also noticed that it happened at the very lowest and saddest times in his life.

This really bothered him and he questioned the Lord about it.

"Lord, You said that once I decided to follow You, You'd walk with me all the way. But I have noticed that during the most troublesome times in my life, there is only one set of footprints. I don't understand why when I needed You most, You would leave me."

The Lord replied, "My son, My precious child, I love you and would never leave you. During your times of trial and suffering, when you saw only one set of footprints, it was then that I carried you."

- Author Unknown

1

DISEASE

"Ma-lady" Awaits

Disease is defined by *Webster's Dictionary* as "an unhealthy condition in an organism caused by infection, poisoning, etc." Affected by economic conditions, wars and natural disasters, disease has always played a role in the history of our societies. Disease can be classified into two very broad groups: infectious and non-infectious. Infectious diseases can spread from one person to another and are caused by microscopic organisms that invade the body. Non-infectious diseases are not communicable from person to person and do not have, or are not known to involve, infectious agents. Many illnesses are acute, coming on suddenly and lasting for no more than several days. Other diseases such as arthritis, lupus, and multiple sclerosis are chronic, intermittently persisting for long intervals.

Dr. Ronald Finn, chief consultant of the Royal Liverpool Hospital in Liverpool, England, divides illness or disease into "congenital, degenerative and environmental. Environmental illness is subdivided into infectious and non-infectious, i.e. chemical, physical...

Many of the common diseases are due to interactions between these groups. Thus a very common cause of disease is due to the interaction of an environmental agent in a genetically susceptible individual. Congenital and degenerative disease is difficult to treat but the removal of an environmental cause is theoretically much easier and effective, providing irrevocable damage has not already occurred."

Every disease has certain characteristic effects on the body. These effects are called symptoms and may include, fever, pain, inflammation, dizziness, nausea, fatigue, and rashes. Symptoms offer important clues that direct people to the type of remedy necessary, which may include the use of natural remedies or visiting your physician.

Disease is generated by a combination of circumstances both inside and outside the body. In our age of rapid industrialization, highly polluted environments, modern technology, and the rapid pace of modern society, a vast number of factors can initiate disease.

Due to the work of scientists, public health officials, and other members of the medical community, once devastating diseases such as smallpox and diphtheria have been virtually eradicated and many diseases that once proved fatal are now treated successfully.

However new diseases, such as AIDS (Acquired Immune Deficiency Syndrome), are causing death to thousands of people. So-called "diseases of choice," such as drug and alcohol abuse, poor eating habits, and lack of exercise are ruining society. Continuous air travel in the United States and abroad increases the risk of disease transmission. Importation and exportation of food greatly increases the risk of disease contamination as well.

Infectious diseases are caused by microscopic organisms known as germs or pathogens. Pathogens that infect humans include a wide variety of bacteria, viruses, fungi, protozoan, and parasitic worms. These pathogens can cause cholera, diphtheria, leprosy, pneumonia, strep throat, tuberculosis, and typhoid fever, just to name a few.

Infectious diseases are spread from one person to another by direct contact. Leaving one host through body openings, mucous membranes, and skin wounds and entering the second host through similar channels. An example is moisture droplets spread by a cough or a sneeze. Your mother's sound advice to always cover your mouth or nose when sneezing or coughing tends to make even more sense in this age of increasing illnesses.

Viruses are tens or hundreds of times smaller than bacteria and are able to survive and reproduce in the living cells of a host. Once a virus invades a living cell it directs the cell to make new virus particles, which are released into the surrounding tissues, seeking new cells to infect. Human diseases caused by viruses include mumps, measles, influenza, rabies, hepatitis, smallpox, AIDS, and certain types of cancers. Viruses can be found on any object being contacted by an infectious person. Bacteria that may initiate gonorrhea and syphilis are transmitted during sexual contact. Still other pathogens involve an intermediary carrier, such as an insect.

Fungi are a varied group of generally small organisms that get their food from organic matter. They germinate from reproductive cells called spores, which often have a thick, resistant outer coat that protects against unfavorable environmental conditions. Due to this protective coating, the spores are very tolerant of extreme external conditions adding to the difficulty of treating fungal infections. An example would be the observance of thick, yellow and brittle, finger and toenails of many individuals with fungal infections.

Some fungi are external parasites causing skin conditions such as athlete's foot, ringworm, and jock itch. Fungi invading internal tissues play host to yeast that infect the genital and the intestinal tract. Several fungi species can cause a certain type of pneumonia.

Protozoans are single-celled, animal-like organisms that live in moist environments. The most known pathogenic protozoans are the species that cause malaria, an infectious disease responsible for over 2 million deaths each year. Other protozoans can cause giardiasis and toxoplasmosis.

Parasitic flatworms, including tapeworms, live in the intestines of host organisms. They have a ribbon-like body that may be up to 30 feet in length, depending on the species. Flatworms have been known to cause several serious diseases.

Roundworms are small, tube-like worms that are pointed at both ends. Species that infect human intestines include pinworms, hookworms, and threadworms. A roundworm known as trichinella spiralis can invade human muscle tissue triggering a disease called trichinosis.

Non-infectious diseases include two of the leading killers in the United States, heart disease and cancer. Non-infectious illnesses include disorders such as arthritis, Alzheimer's disease, and Parkinson's disease. All of these diseases involve the breakdown of tissue and loss of bodily function.

Environmental factors play critical roles in numerous non-infectious diseases. Exposure to carbon monoxide can have long-term effects on the heart and vision. Lead can impair mental abilities and increase blood pressure. Long-term exposure to coal and asbestos predisposes people to respiratory diseases. Mercury-amalgam fillings in teeth can add to the total body overload of heavy metal causing havoc throughout the whole body.

Addiction to various substances such as tobacco or alcohol can lead to many diseases. It is well known that these substances may cause lung cancer, bladder cancer, heart disease, liver disease, brain damage and nutritional disorders.

¤¤¤

Hereditary diseases such as Sickle Cell Anemia and Huntington's disease are caused by mutated genes inherited from one or both parents. Certain other diseases, such as diabetes, hypertension, and some types of cancer often run in families, suggesting that heredity may play a role in their development. Allergies, which are increasing in epidemic numbers in the United States, can also be inherited.

Congenital diseases, or birth defects, are disorders that are present at birth. Some are hereditary; others develop while a baby is in its mother's uterus or during the process of delivery. For example, if the mother contracts german measles, or rubella, during the early stages of pregnancy, her child may be born with heart defects, eye cataracts, deafness, or mental retardation. The use of alcohol during pregnancy can cause Fetal Alcohol Syndrome, characterized by mental and physical retardation. Fetal Alcohol Syndrome is growing in rapid numbers in the world today!

Immunological diseases occur when the immune system malfunctions. The most common types of immunological diseases are allergies and autoimmune diseases. Autoimmune diseases develop when the immune system goes awry and attacks the body's own tissues. Examples are lupus, rheumatoid arthritis, and juvenile-onset diabetes.

Immune deficiency diseases develop when the immune system becomes weakened resulting in more frequent or severe infections. Genetic abnormalities, illness, injury, and the use of strong drugs such as those used in chemotherapy, exposure to toxic heavy metals or chemicals, or malnutrition are just a few of the sources that may damage the immune system. Old age is a foe to the immune system. The older adults become, the higher the chance of having a weakened immune system. A case of pneumonia is no match for a strong immune system, whereas for a person with a weakened immune system, pneumonia could prove fatal. Stress, whether caused by foods, chemicals, toxins, or interpersonal problems, place a load on the body which can weaken the immune system.

Deficiency diseases result from low amounts of necessary body nutrients. Examples include scurvy, caused by a deficiency of Vitamin C; pellagra, caused by a deficiency of niacin; and osteoporosis, caused at least in part by a lack of calcium in the proper form. Deficiency diseases are most prevalent in poverty or war stricken areas of the world, where malnutrition is widespread. They are also found in more affluent nations where food is plentiful, but people's food choices or behavior do not provide well-rounded nutrition, thus resulting in the general breakdown of health leading to disease, suffering, and eventually, death. Chronic illness in the United States today serves as a prime example of deficiency diseases.

Psychological diseases are on the increase. Depression and anxiety seem to be common place in today's society. Illness is a natural expression of occurrences inside the body. It is futile to treat illness with superficial drugs which are designed to suppress the problem. Each person needs to examine their own health identifying their current physical, mental, and emotional states. Let us rebalance our diets, our lifestyles, our lives. Every person has the potential for good health. Fighting disease requires dedication to a chosen lifestyle and the desire to have a healthy body as a reward.

The mind is immensely powerful and the relationship between mind and body should never be underestimated. All thoughts and emotions affect every cell in the body and physiologically manifest themselves in various forms. Many diseases have their roots in the emotional health of their victims.

~

MOTIVATIONAL TIP

Although we live in a world of disease, the fear of contracting a serious ailment can be minimized. Adherence to the steps outlined in this book will decrease the chances of disease. Begin taking measures now to increase your opportunity of dying peacefully at a ripe old age, quietly in your sleep, pain free, through the natural aging process, without a disease ridden and suffering body.

~

"Real knowledge is to know the extent of ones ignorance."

- Confucius

2

NUTRITIONAL DEFICIENCIES

A Hungry People

It is a well-known fact that the general American diet is nutritionally deficient. Several factors are responsible for this fact.

For decades, agricultural practices have been depleting minerals from the soil, thus compromising soil health. If it isn't in the soil, it's not in the food! Over the past fifty years, there has been a steady decline in the mineral content of soil and thus, in whole foods.

Other factors that affect nutritional deficiencies include premature harvesting, extended storage and shipping of crops. Food additives and food preparation can also cause food degradation. Considering all factors, most food delivered to the dinner table is void of many health building nutrients.

If we are to consume more nutritious foods, we must take steps to ensure that they grow in nutrient rich soil. The foods should ripen on the vine and be delivered to your home the fastest way possible to prevent nutrient loss. These foods should be prepared in their most natural state.

The best way to accomplish this is to grow your own food in your backyard. We must utilize our gardens and greenhouses to ensure our family is receiving nutrient rich foods, promoting good health.

Grow your own fruits and vegetables in the summer season. Soil should be fertilized and cultivated on a yearly basis. Fresh food should be taken directly from the vine, washed and placed on the table in a raw state. If you do not have space or time to plant your own, most areas have a farmer's cooperative agency or organic farmers that sell fresh fruits and vegetables at reasonable prices.

Growing and preserving your own food for year-round use would be a huge step in the right direction. It is much work but well worth the effort. Preserving your own food is not always cost effective but is definitely health effective. Remember fresh is best, frozen and dried is next best, followed by canned (in glass) foods.

If you spend time preparing the ground, planting the seeds, cultivating, weeding, watering and protecting your garden, make sure you also take the time to preserve your produce correctly. There are many wonderful and helpful books in print that can assist you in doing this. It is extremely disappointing to realize that you have over processed your jars or haven't done something correctly to seal your jars. Although frozen foods have more nutrients than canned you should realize that if the electric power is interrupted for an extended period of time, you could lose all your frozen produce. It is wise to preserve your foods utilizing various methods. Remember the saying, "Don't put all your eggs in one basket."

Knowing that no preservatives or chemicals are being consumed provides a soothing thought. Remember to use herbs in seasoning soups, vegetables, and meats. Herbs enhance the flavor of food and are a healthy and nutritious alternative. Sea salt or kosher salt is also a needed staple in every kitchen to not only enhance taste but to improve health. Remember, salt is an alkalizing food and is very healing to the body. Do not buy salt from your local grocery store as it is usually treated with dextrose and other chemicals. You will find sea salt or kosher salt at reputable whole foods stores.

Due to the lack of nutrients in the foods we eat, many people take a broad-spectrum multi-vitamin/mineral supplement. It is essential to educate yourself concerning the quality of these vitamins. Many are of poor quality, improperly balanced, composed of many synthetic compounds, and are not properly assimilated or absorbed. There are high quality vitamin and mineral supplements available; however, you are unlikely to find them at your local grocery store. Rather, locate your supplements at reputable health food stores or better yet at credible companies that are continually researching and improving their products (see Life Changing Products).

Many people's immune systems are compromised to the point that a multi-vitamin/mineral supplement is not enough to correct the deficiency. It is necessary to receive a complete physical, conducted by a licensed physician who understands natural health and nutrition.

After receiving the results of the necessary testing, your physician will determine your deficiencies and will provide you with information on what supplements you will need to take to eliminate these deficiencies. It is vital to get products that can be properly assimilated by the body. A vitamin or mineral that is not absorbed into the body is of no value.

Research your needs before investing in any supplements! There are many good health books and manuals that will help you assess your symptoms and the likelihood of deficiencies. Combine this with the guidance given to you by your healthcare provider (see Resource Guide and Bibliography).

Educate yourself. It is your body and your health.

You can eat all the proper foods and take balanced and quality supplements to meet your deficiencies but if your digestion is poor, your efforts will prove futile. The old adage, "you are what you eat" is inaccurate in my opinion. "You are what you absorb" is a more accurate statement.

Digestion refers to the mechanical and chemical process of the breakdown of food from large to small molecules. Assimilation refers to the transport of nutrients across membranes of the gastrointestinal tract into the bloodstream and lymph system, where eventually they are carried into cells throughout the body for utilization.

The gastrointestinal tract has been wonderfully designed with glands and organs that on demand, secrete specialized fluids and perform intricate churning actions. This process transforms food into a state that the intestinal lining can then absorb. The whole digestive tract is lined with millions of goblet cells that produce mucus to lubricate organs and protect the mucosa from mechanical and chemical injury. However, injury, imbalance, and malfunction seem inevitable for many Americans.

Of great concern, are the chronic health problems of children in the United States today. These numbers are increasing in epidemic proportions. If you have children or have children in your care, do not neglect the seemingly trivial symptoms they display. Just like a new car, children should be running at peak performance. They are young, they are new, and should not be malfunctioning. Strive to maintain their immune systems at the highest level possible. Refined sugars, harmful fats and environmental toxins are aging the internal organs of our youth at alarming rates!

The first phase of digestion actually takes place before you take your first bite of food. Intricate neurological and hormonal communications occur between the brain and the digestive system. These signals, triggered by the odors of food, the anticipation of eating and the sensation of hunger, prepare the digestive organs for their work.

If you are hungry, relaxed, and able to enjoy food, these hormonal communications take place. If you are tense, anxious, angry, or excited when eating, these signals are not properly communicated. It is better not to eat than to eat during times of inner turmoil.

Obviously, if you are always tense, angry, or hurried you must still eat. If this is the case, ensure your meals are extremely nutritious and small. It is vital you do not overload your system when one of the aforementioned conditions exists.

Chewing is the next stage in the digestion process. If food is not thoroughly broken down by the mechanical act of chewing, often only the outer surfaces of the large food morsels will be exposed to your digestive secretions. In such a condition, you might feel satisfied, but the food in your stomach is not necessarily being metabolized so that nutrients are reaching your cells. The undigested food reaching your colon will trigger a state of toxicity.

Chewing thoroughly is a major factor in good digestion and assimilation. You should eat slowly and take small bites, making sure to chew food thoroughly, until it is of a creamy substance before swallowing. You should not feel individual pieces of food prior to swallowing. If you are unable to chew your food then it is better to blend your food in a processor, making it more digestible.

As mentioned in Chapter 19, it is important not to drink liquids with your meals. Water or beverages confuse the stomach into thinking that this liquid is a digestive enzyme, thereby hindering the digestion process. It also dilutes the digestive liquids, thus requiring more hydrochloric acid, which can cause further problems.

Do not eat between meals. Any food eaten after the digestion process has started begins the process all over again, thus leaving partially digested food to ferment, causing terrible digestive problems.

Excessive physical activity is also not recommended immediately following a meal. Your digestive system uses a great amount of energy to assimilate the food you have eaten. Muscular activity will shift your body's focus and circulation away from your digestive system toward your muscles, leaving the digestive system on hold and unable to do its job well. A short walk, however, soon after eating can actually enhance the process. Whatever you do, try not to lie down, sleep, or slouch in your easy chair. This goes against the digestive process.

Regular bowel elimination is a requirement of good health. If the lower part of the gastrointestinal tract becomes sluggish (constipation), the digestive functions farther up the tract become impaired. You may have a sluggish colon even if you are having one or more eliminations per day. Ideally within one hour of ingesting food, your body should have a bowel elimination.

¤¤¤

There are many interrelated components to successful digestion and assimilation:

- Being hungry and relaxed for meals.

- Consuming 80 percent alkaline and 20 percent acidic foods.

- Chewing well.

- Selecting healthful, whole foods.

- Eating clean non-chemically treated foods.

- Eating at least 75 percent raw foods. (This amount of raw foods may not work well with all individuals, especially throughout the winter months and may need to be adjusted accordingly.)

- Eating sensible portions and at the right times.

- Not drinking with your meals.

- Proper food combinations.

- Being aware of the importance of bowel elimination.

- Adequate enzymes.

¤¤¤

In addition to the above, it is also important to identify and avoid food allergens. The need to identify and treat bacterial infections (i.e. heliobacter pylori), parasites, and yeast infections is also very important.

The digestive tract is one of the more abused systems of our bodies. A multi-million-dollar industry has evolved to treat such digestive disorders as indigestion, constipation, diarrhea, coated tongue, bad breath and body odor. Although these ailments are irritating, they are pale in comparison to the conditions that may attack your body later as a result of neglecting your digestive system. Conditions such as fatigue, hypoglycemia, anemia, arthritis, osteoporosis, hypertension and arteriosclerosis render the body more susceptible to infections and cancer. With this knowledge firmly planted in your minds, you should now realize that immediate action is required if any of the above symptoms are present.

~

MOTIVATIONAL TIPS

Proper digestion and absorption of nutrients are paramount to maintaining your good health and well being. Make a decision today to begin the process in preventing chronic illnesses. It is never too early to begin.

Your diet should consist of a variety of foods. However do limit each meal to no more than three or four different foods.

Make every meal exciting. Ensure your dinner table looks appetizing to your family! Serve a colorful raw salad of fresh vegetables first. Do not serve cooked foods until the salads are finished.

Experiment in using flavorful herbs to make your dishes delectable.

Treat yourself to a new cookbook. With the growing interest in nutrition and whole foods, you will find a wide selection to fit every need (see Resource Guide).

Remember, eating healthy foods rejuvenates the life force by supplying the body with multiple anti-aging nutrients. You will not only feel great, you will look great too!

~

"Problems cannot be solved at the same level of awareness that created them."
- Albert Einstein

Your Thoughts

3

pH BALANCE

Acid vs. Alkaline

The human body is three-fourths alkaline. Our blood is slightly alkaline and our urine is slightly acidic in nature. A diet too heavily dependent on acidic foods causes a blood electrolyte imbalance. In order to balance the blood electrolyte, the body uses stored alkaline minerals. An acidic diet robs the system of alkaline minerals such as sodium, potassium, magnesium and calcium, leaving us prone to many degenerative diseases (ex: gallstones, kidney stones, gout and osteoporosis). Clinical signs of acidosis are headache, slowness in responding to questions, hand tremor when extending arms, confusion, drowsiness, nausea, vomiting, tremor, rapid heart rate, increased breathing, and ultimately coma. The stress on our kidneys and cells has a depleting effect on our immune system leaving us prone to colds, viral infections and cancers.

Normally, bile produced by the liver, eradicates parasites at all stages of development in a healthy organism. Bile neutralizes the acidic environment of food.

It also aids in preparing the food for digestion and absorption within the small intestine.

The pH balance of the body could play a key role in disease. What we eat truly can make a difference in how our body responds to illness. An overabundance of foods high in acid (chronic acidosis) permits an excessive load on the liver's bile production and detoxification. During this process, the body searches other sources for neutralizing minerals. The process of finding and utilizing these necessary minerals depletes other regions of the body. When a proper pH balance is present, Vitamin B-12 is produced. Due to the body's difficulty assimilating ingested B-12, people lacking in B-12 are usually given a semi-annual injection.

Chronic acidosis promotes the formation of gallstones and liver exhaustion. The result is eventual overrun by parasites that can lead to cancer and other diseases. This topic is further discussed in Chapter 11. Having a proper pH diet and healthy intestinal flora promotes an environment where parasites cannot thrive (see Life Changing Products). The body can then properly assimilate calcium, magnesium, potassium, and sodium minerals.

Acidity in the stomach is not necessarily related to chronic acidosis. HCL (Hydrochloric Acid) in the stomach is required for digestion. What is of concern, however, is the pH level in the ash left behind following digestion. In fact, high levels of acid in the body actually inhibit the production of stomach acids. The absorption of B-12 is dependent upon a high level of HCL in the stomach. A diet high in alkaline assures us the body will absorb the B-12. When the body's pH is too acidic, the body's response is to compensate by secreting less acidic fluids and a shortage of proper stomach acid is the result.

When the body has utilized the readily available supplies of sodium and calcium, it will steal calcium from bones in an attempt to neutralize the acidosis. Because the body cannot leach enough calcium to meet the pH demands of the blood electrolyte, the liver begins manufacturing ammonia to compensate. This ammonia solvent is harmful to the body and promotes the growth of parasites.

High ammonia content is common to most cancer patients. Their bodies are attempting to neutralize the acidosis. The high pH reading in their bodies is due to the level of ammonia being produced, because of an improper diet. Anyone visiting a cancer ward will notice a distinct smell of ammonia.

The body will produce the strongest pH it can to obtain the nutrients from food. A pH of 6.0 and below will cause the body to begin experiencing acidic digestive symptoms (gas, bloating, and loose stools). A pH of 7.0 and above leads to alkaline (or weakening) digestive symptoms, marked by slow digestion and constipation (which is really eliminating less than two to three times a day).

The proper pH balance would be near the halfway mark at 6.5.

Poor digestion signified by a weak saliva (pH 6.0 and below), indicates a need to eat more because we digest less, explaining many people's current eating and weight dilemma. The digestive strength is gone and we are continually hungry because our bodies are not getting the nutrients from our food. This in turn affects our health and immune system, as we become more and more deficient. Although the pH test in medicine is well known and documented, it appears the relationship between the pH

tion, and eliminative systems are overlooked by
lical practitioners. Consequently implications
l to diet and deficiencies are mostly ignored.

When our digestion is too acidic, our foods move through us too quickly and are not fully absorbed, thus leading to deficiencies as well. Prepare to make better food choices by learning which foods are acidic and which are alkaline. These foods are discussed in the next chapter. The key is moderation in consuming acidic foods. It is up to each of us to research and determine a diet that gives us the greatest feeling of well-being, maintains overall health, and can be incorporated into our lifestyle with ease. A diet that we do not view as deprivation, but one we embrace with absolute determination and enthusiasm.

~

MOTIVATIONAL TIP

Immediately begin taking responsibility for your health! Visit your local pharmacy and request a roll of Nitrazine paper. It usually is dispensed in rolls measuring 1-inch by 15-feet and costs approximately $35.00. This may seem expensive but it lasts for a very long time. Place a small piece in your month before eating in the morning and then forty-five minutes after lunch and dinner. The paper will immediately begin turning color. Match the color of your test results with the color shown on the dispenser. Optimum range is 6.5. As you get closer to 6.5, the need and frequency of this test will decrease.

~

"You must be the change you wish to see in the world."

- Mahatma Gandhi

Your Thoughts

4

FOOD COMBINING

Watermelon & Oreo's Don't Mix

Now let's look at some of the foods that will enable us to maintain a proper pH balance. As a general rule we can say that most unfired (unchanged by cooking i.e. heat and microwave), living and unprocessed vegetables and fruits are alkaline forming. Most, if not all, processed, cooked and fried foods are acid forming. All dairy products, meat, fish, poultry, sweets (except raw honey), and unsprouted flour products are acid forming foods. An acid environment is a perfect breeding ground for parasites and degenerative diseases.

The list would be too extensive to categorize all foods into acid/alkaline groups. Please use the above information as a general rule and perform your own research on identification of specific foods. You will find some sources may list a particular food as acid while another may list the same food as alkaline. This is due to the food being close to the middle of the acid/alkaline spectrum. Thus, the author chose one class or the other for identification purposes. Listed below is just one example of the many acid/alkaline food charts that are available to us:

¤¤¤

Fruits
Acid
Cranberries
Pomegranates
Strawberries
Sour Fruits

Alkaline
Apples
Bananas
Citrus Fruits
Dates
Grapes
Cherries
Peaches
Pears
Plums
Papaya
Mangoes
Pineapple
Raspberries
Blackberries
Huckleberries
Elderberries
Boysenberries

Grains
Acid
Brown Rice
Barley
Wheat
Oats
Rye
Breads
Buckwheat
Corn

Alkaline
Millet
Sprouted Grains

Sugars
Acid
Brown Sugar
White Sugar
Milk Sugar
Cane Sugar
Malt Syrup
Maple Syrup
Molasses

Nuts
Acid
Cashews
Walnuts
Filberts
Peanuts
Pecans
Macadamia

Alkaline
Almonds
Brazil

Sugars
Alkaline
Honey

Fruits (cont.)
Alkaline
Persimmons
Apricots
Olives
Coconut
Figs
Raisins
Melons

Meats/Dairy
Acid
All Meats
Fish
Fowl
Eggs
Cheese
Milk
Yogurt
Butter

Seeds
Acid
Pumpkin
Sesame
Sunflower
Chia
Flax

Alkaline
Sprouted Seeds

Beans/Peas
Acid
Lentils
Navy
Kidney

Alkaline
Soybeans
Limas
Sprouted Beans

Oils
Acid
Nut Oils
Butter
Cream

Alkaline
Olive Oil
Soy
Sesame
Sunflower
Corn
Safflower
Cottonseed
Margarine

Alkaline:
All vegetables are alkaline (includes starchy vegetables such as, potatoes, squash and parsnips).

¤¤¤

After cooking foods, they may change from alkaline to acid, as is the case of the much-loved tomato. Prior to cooking the tomato, it is an alkaline food. However, if you set yourself down to a big plate of pasta smothered in thick, rich tomato sauce along with a slice of garlic bread and a glass of milk, you just consumed a huge amount of acidic foods.

Our most alkaline food is sodium. Sodium is alkaline to the alimentary tract and is capable of turning around a bad case of acidosis. The alkaline principle in food can cure most diseases without doctors or drugs. Celery is full of sodium and therefore is a powerful alkaline food.

Personal diets should consist of a daily regimen of 80 percent alkaline and 20 percent acid. Most Americans have this totally reversed! Also, a ratio of 75 percent raw and 25 percent cooked should be a daily occurrence unless you are unable to tolerate such a high percentage of raw foods. Are you beginning to understand where diseases begin?

A discussion of food combining is necessary, allowing a better understanding of combinations providing the best opportunity for the proper assimilation of foods by the body.

Different foods in different food groups require vastly different enzymes for proper digestion. If you do not observe the proper food combination rules, then putrefication, fermentation and constipation are certain results. Symptoms may appear that would suggest the existence of diseases such as diverticulitis and colitis to more serious manifestations such as cysts, tumors and cancer.

The routine diet of a person will ultimately determine the difference between good and bad health. So, that juicy cheeseburger on a soft white bun, and a large order of fries, preceded by an appetizer and a beer, followed with a rich desert and coffee is just about the worst kind of food and food combination possible. And yet, from a nutritionist's point of view you had a portion of all food groups and probably met most of your Recommended Daily Allowances!

Another example is the traditional Thanksgiving meal. After eating, many people get tired and lethargic because of the load placed on their system. Their body is working overtime trying to digest these particular food combinations as well as the high fat content of the meal. The body is placed under such strain that we have no energy left for anything else. That is why we find so many people relaxing in their easy chairs after the holiday dinner. Of course, the tryptophan in the turkey also serves to relax us!

Let's take a look at fruits and what three different categories they fall into. Citrus fruits reduce acidity and cause alkalinity. Citrus fruits, when broken down, release an alkaline ash, which develops an alkaline condition in the body. Sometimes these fruits stir up the acids so rapidly that their effect is considered to be a bad one.

If the eating of these fruits causes minor distress, it is most likely caused by the cleansing of the body. A mistake is probably made distinguishing cleansing from disease. If this type of distress is prevalent, seek advice from a physician experienced in natural medicine and nutrition.

In general, fruits should be eaten in a natural harmony. Oranges, grapefruits, tangerines, lemons and limes all have the same kind of seeds, and combine perfectly. You can also mix these with other acid fruits like cranberries, and strawberries but since they have differing seeds the combination is less than perfect.

Melons should <u>always</u> be eaten alone. There is no more disagreeable surprise for your stomach than to eat watermelon with another type of food. Melons require a special enzymic action, which other foods inhibit. If you eat melon, eat it alone or leave it alone.

Any fruit or combination thereof should be eaten without any additives, such as cream, sugar, or chocolate. Fruit already contains sugar. You do not need to add sugar to sugar!

Try this routine!

Immediately after waking in the morning, drink a large glass of warm water with a twist of fresh lemon. Approximately thirty to sixty minutes later consume some fruit. Fruit has a cleansing effect on the body and morning is when you are most toxic. Fruit also tends to digest rapidly therefore bringing on a movement of elimination. This is an excellent schedule to begin and maintain.

It is better to have a serving of one or two types of fruit than a serving of several types of fruit. The simpler the food combination the easier the assimilation process. While the human body is an incredible machine, it is essential proper care is taken to ensure a healthy body. The less stress to our systems the better.

CONSIDERATIONS

- Various foods are digested in different areas of the body in different ways. Starches begin to break down in the mouth when they mix with enzymes in the saliva.

- Protein should be eaten first so that the HCL (Hydrochloric Acid) can work on them immediately. You can then eat vegetables, but do not eat any fruit. Fruits cause an alkaline substance to be excreted, which inhibits protein and starch digestion.

- Do not drink any beverages with your meal. Drinking during or within one- and one-half to- two hours after a meal dilutes the HCL in your stomach, which will inhibit or slow down digestion.

- As food leaves the stomach and goes into the duodenum (upper part of the small intestine), it is acted upon by many different enzymes secreted by the pancreas, according to the type of food the body is ingesting. At this point bile is received from the liver through the gallbladder to aid digestion. Because of this marvelous and intricate digestive process, it is better to watch combinations of food at any one meal. For example, high acid and low acid foods should not be combined, nor should fruits and vegetables.

- Protein foods can be combined with vegetables; starches can be combined with vegetables to produce a fair balance.

- Tobacco, coffee, chocolate, sugar and most other things we crave are acid forming and should be avoided completely.

- Most drugs are also acid forming.

- Phosphorus and sulfur act as buffers to maintain pH balance. Sulfur can be taken in supplement form (ie. MSM), or consumed by eating sulfur containing foods such as garlic and onion.

- Herbs that can be used to remedy acidosis are elder bark, hops and willow.

~

MOTIVATIONAL TIP

Some people are very sick and their lives are in jeopardy. They are forced to be motivated to change their diet immediately. If you can do this I commend you. However, realize there is much to learn and adjust to in changing your diet. Do the very best you can and continue to research and learn. Do not be too judgmental or hard on yourself. If you fail, pick yourself up and continue forward. Remember, it took years to get sick and it will take time to regain your health.

~

"Fall seven times, stand up eight."
- Japanese Proverb

5

ENZYMES

Break Me Down

We have discussed the importance of proper nutrition, the type of foods that will provide this nutrition, and how the teeth aid in digestion by cutting and masticating the food. We have discussed acid vs. alkaline foods, what foods combine well and what foods should never be combined. However if the body does not assimilate the food we eat, then all of this information is useless.

Within our diets, enzymes are required to break down and utilize the various vitamins and nutrients. They are used in all vital body functions. Many people experience a shortage of enzymes from eating too much processed and/or fast-foods, as all of these foods are bankrupt of vital enzymes.

Enzymes are perhaps our most important nutrients. Enzymes are responsible for nearly every facet of life and health. As we age, there is a slow and gradual decrease in the enzyme content of our bodies. We must have a constant enzyme supply which requires continual replacement of enzymes.

Enzymes are unique proteins, which are essential components of over 90 trillion cells, composing every tissue of every organ in our body. Without enzymes, very few of our essential metabolic processes would take place. They regulate the digestion of our food, the production of energy, the production of hormones, the production of other body secretions, and the destruction of foreign substances.

Raw fruits and vegetables are important to the diet, as cooking foods destroys many enzymes. Fruits and vegetables must be fresh, as enzymes are very active chemically and do not remain stable in the produce as it ages. Keeping the produce cool is also important, due to the fact enzymes are depleted more quickly at warmer temperatures.

Many people that suffer from stomach upset, heartburn, acid indigestion, bloating, gas, nausea, burping, diarrhea, constipation, hiatal hernia, gastritis or ulcers have enzyme deficiencies.

There are four food enzymes required for bringing about optimal digestion and assimilation of nutrients, reducing stomach acidity, restoring appetite, and assisting in balancing the body's natural pH (acid/base) balance.

¤¤¤

Amylase for Carbohydrates

A deficiency in amylase enzymes can cause poor digestion of carbohydrates, sugars and starches. Symptoms may include:

- Infections, abscesses, and inflammation.

- Skin conditions, including eczema, psoriasis, hives, dermatitis, and herpes.

- Asthma and emphysema (may be aggravated by amylase deficiency).

Cellulase for Fiber

Poor digestion of fiber or plant substances can be caused by a deficiency in cellulase enzymes. Poor digestion may also cause a person to experience Malabsorption Syndrome. Symptoms may include:

- Frequent gas, pain, and bloating.

- Impaired absorption of nutrients, vitamins, and minerals.

- Increased sugar, dairy, gluten (wheat, oats, rye, barley) intolerance or allergy, which can be associated with celiac disease, or Crohn's disease.

Lipase for Fats

Lipase enzymes digest fats and fat-soluble vitamins. Many people deficient in lipase enzymes have a tendency towards high cholesterol, high triglycerides, and may have difficulty with losing weight, diabetes or heart disease. Poor digestion of fats can cause a deficiency in EFA (Essential Fatty Acids). EFA deliver lubrication and moisture to the skin, joints, and cardiovascular system. This assists in preventing dryness, inflammations, and heart disease. EFA bind oxygen to hemoglobin, increasing oxygenation and circulation throughout the whole body.

Protease for Protein

Poor digestion can be due to a deficiency of protease enzymes or an imbalance in pH. This poor digestion can create a variety of symptoms including:

- Poor recovery time after exercise.

- Hypoglycemia (blood sugar imbalances, sugar cravings, or mood swings).

- Poor utilization of calcium and magnesium. These minerals must bond with amino acids (proteins) to be fully assimilated for bone strength and calming the nervous system. This helps to prevent osteoporosis, arthritis, anxiety, irritability, and insomnia.

- Loss of muscle mass.

¤¤¤

To summarize: when enzyme levels in the body diminish and when dietary levels decrease, the stage is set for the development of poor health and possible weight gain. Choosing a diet containing high levels of raw fruits and vegetables and supplementing with high potency enzymes only makes good health sense (see Life Changing Products).

~

MOTIVATIONAL TIPS

Today, begin eating a plate of fresh organically grown fruits or vegetables. Start taking a high potency enzyme with <u>each</u> meal. Continue this process and within a few weeks, many of your digestive problems will disappear. Keep a diary of your symptoms and the date you begin these new eating habits. You will be pleasantly surprised!

Please feel free to contact me for resources providing high quality enzymes and whole foods fruit, vegetable and grain supplements. When eating the proper amount of fruits and vegetables each day is not possible, these whole food supplements will provide you the nutrition your body requires. These foods are also backed by scientific research and study.

~

"Character cannot be developed in ease of quiet. Only through experience of trial and suffering can the soul be strengthened, ambition inspired, and success achieved."
- Helen Keller

Your Thoughts

6

JUICING

Your Daily Blood Transfusion

Fresh juice provides us with minerals, vitamins, essential fatty acids, carbohydrates, proteins and much more. Regular juicing may be one of the keys to good health, as it is an important source of raw food, which contains chlorophyll and phytonutrients (nutrients from plant foods).

The phytochemicals that researchers have uncovered are changing the way we think about food, especially fruits and vegetables. For example, broccoli contains a substance that may prevent breast cancer. Citrus fruits have substances that make it easier for your body to remove carcinogens, thus decreasing the chance of developing cancer. Grapes contain a phytochemical that appears to protect each cell's DNA from damage. Similarly, a number of green vegetables contain phytochemicals that seem to offer protection against cancer-causing substances. Among the foods on the list that appear to have cancer preventing phytochemicals are bok choy, broccoli, brussels sprouts, cabbage, cauliflower, carrots, collards, kale, kohlrabi, mustard greens, rutabaga, turnip greens, red beets, peppers, garlic, onions, leeks, and chives.

It is never too late to start juicing! Juices can flush toxins from your body, are good for your weight, heart, circulation and overall well being. They contain no saturated fats or added sodium and can be helpful in lowering your cholesterol. They are a real boost for your immune system and should be enjoyed <u>each</u> and <u>every day</u>.

You will find that as you juice fruits and vegetables their goodness is released from the fiber and you are able to drink their highly concentrated nutrients, which are then able to enter your bloodstream very quickly. Of course fiber is essential to good health, so be sure to continue eating raw fruits and vegetables. In fact, as you become more creative with your juicing, I would advise drinking 80 percent of the juice and add back in some of the pulp to the remaining 20 percent and consume immediately.

Most bottled juices on the market today have had valuable nutrients removed through the bottling process. Heat destroys the enzymes, which assist you in assimilating their nutrients. If you make your own juice and drink it fresh, you will have control over the quality of the fruits and vegetables you are consuming as well as saving money.

The best time to juice is in the morning. After a whole night of sleep your body not only needs to be lubricated with pure water, but also needs to begin cleansing toxins and rebuilding cells. Juicing cleanses as well as rebuilds.

Juice should be consumed as soon as it has been extracted and should be sipped and swished around in the mouth before swallowing. This will encourage the pancreas to react and create enzymes, which will enhance the assimilation process. Never gulp your ju experience stomach cramps or nausea.

If you have never juiced before, you s using vegetables that you enjoy eating wł cucumber, celery and carrot are the most ʋₒₗₑᵣₐᵦₗₑ ᵥₑ ₐₗₗ vegetable juices. As you become accustomed to the taste begin to juice leafy green vegetables, like kale, wheat or barley grasses, lettuces, chards, broccoli, and cabbage. The chlorophyll in the plants will react to your system like a blood transfusion. You will immediately start noticing an increase in energy. Include beets in your juice at least twice per week, as they are a great liver and kidney cleanser. Beets, both leaf and root are excellent blood builders. Add fresh ginger root for a unique and healthy treat.

Begin your juicing slowly, taking only a few ounces per day. If you start out consuming too much at one time, you may experience nausea or other digestive problems as your body begins the cleansing process. Work up to at least 32 ounces of fresh juice each day.

Although, fruit juices may taste better to you than vegetable juices, they should be juiced sparingly due to the high sugar content, which can play havoc on insulin levels. Use these as a treat juice!

Never mix vegetable and fruit juices together. You will see all kinds of concoctions for great tasting juice recipes and while they may taste good, mixing them with each other is not good for the digestive system. They will have difficulty being assimilated and may cause digestive disturbances. Rotate your juices to avoid boredom and becoming allergic to frequently juiced foods.

Whenever possible, use only certified organically grown produce. The real reason behind juicing is not because it is fun or that it will always taste fantastic. We e to build and maintain our health. Therefore, why ice pesticides, insecticides and fungicides along with our fruits and vegetables. If you can't find "certified organic" produce at your local grocery, request the produce manager to begin stocking them. Also encourage friends and family to make the same request for their local markets. Grocers will stock anything that sells!

Purchase a good juicer. Many inexpensive juicers do not separate the pulp and juice well. They also run at high speeds, which creates heat as the juices are extracted, diminishing the nutrient content. If you are going to take juicing seriously, you must invest in a good quality juice extractor (see Life Changing Products).

~

MOTIVATIONAL TIPS

There are many great Internet sites and well written books on the art of juicing. Make a commitment to research for yourself the advantages that juicing fresh "certified organic" fruits and vegetables will make in your overall health.

Keep a journal of how you feel each morning. Note all details. Start juicing tomorrow and continue the routine each day. Note how you have changed physically, emotionally and mentally. You will experience a remarkable difference. One of the first things I noticed was increased energy, an improvement in my complexion and shiny, healthy hair. It will be well worth the extra effort and you will not be able to imagine your life without consuming fresh juices each and every day.

Many people just do not take the time to juice and consume 32 ounces of juice per day and they certainly do not consume the suggested servings of fruits and vegetables per day that is recommended by the National Cancer Institute. When time constraints make regular juicing impossible, it is important that you do not miss out on these vital nutrients. Fruits and vegetables in capsule form will help assist in providing the needed nutrients during these times. Remember, not all products are the same! I have done my homework and have located a company with remarkably high quality products and the scientific research to back them up. Contact me for further information or visit our website.

~

"Look and you will find it - what is unsought is undetected."

- Sophocles

Your Thoughts

7

SPROUTING

Powerhouse Explosion

Sprouting is a foreign word to many people, in today's fast-paced, fast-food society, yet it is one of the most nutritional practices available to improve and maintain your health. Every seed is a plant embryo just waiting for the perfect conditions to break forth into life and germinate into a powerhouse of energy. When a seed meets the right combination of moisture, air and temperature, it will suddenly sprout forth, providing, a cleansing, detoxifying, rebuilding effect on the body. Using sprouts varies the menu, adds bulk, and improves the flavor of many dishes. It is easy and sprouting seeds can help support any family's over-worked budget. As disease and illness run rampant in today's society, sprouting is becoming more and more popular in America, as people search for answers to overcome diseases, as well as those folks looking for ways to prevent illness.

Sprouting has been around for many centuries, dating back to at least 2939 B.C., when first mentioned in a book by the Emperor of China. The Chinese had probably used sprouts for a long time before that, and they are still a very important part of the Chinese cuisine.

There are many reasons for sprouting: Nutritionally, dried seeds, grains, and legumes provide only a small portion of the total nutrients the body requires. However, once sprouted, seeds provide the largest relative amount of nutrients per unit of intake compared to other food sources. Sprouts can aid a body that is consistently exposed to toxic chemicals and is undergoing an immune system decline. They taste delicious, are highly nutritious, improve health, save time and money, are low in calories, give quick energy and are an important addition to the home food storage programs. It is virtually impossible for a family to store enough fresh vegetables to last a long period of time or to have them available in times of extreme duress, whether due to manmade or natural disasters. By sprouting seeds, fresh vegetables are only two to three days away, year-round. Sprouting seeds is also a great way to increase the utility of many types of grains, seeds, and legumes or beans.

Anyone who enjoys raw vegetables and salads will most likely enjoy sprouts. They can also be a great addition to cooked dishes, soups, pancakes, casseroles and breads. It will be rare that you will find a better tasting loaf of bread than one made with sprouted grains or legumes. As with most foods, the nutritional value of sprouts is higher when eaten raw; however, much of the vitamins and minerals remain stable even when included in heated foods. In fact, cooking, baking, and steaming does allow for greater absorption of some foods through increased bioavailability.

In the sprouting process there is a dramatic increase in the vitamin and mineral content of seeds, beans and grains which aid in the development of the seed during its growth process. There is more nourishment contained in a plant's sprout, than at any other time in its life cycle. Often, new nutrients occur where there were none before. Vitamins A, B complex, C, and E are increased sometimes as much as ten times! For example, the dry soybean has no Vitamin C. Dr. Pauline Berry Mack, at the University of Pennsylvania, found after sprouting seeds for 72 hours, that one-half cup of the sprouts contained as much Vitamin C as six glasses of orange juice. Dr. Paul Burkholder, at Yale University, sprouted oats for five days and discovered that the B vitamins had skyrocketed 500 percent; B6 vitamins, 600 percent more; increased folic acid; B1 vitamins, 10 percent more; and B2 vitamins 135 percent more than before sprouting. Sprouted oats also have 600 percent more C vitamins than unsprouted oats. Because the enzymes are all active in these raw foods, they can be easily assimilated into the body.

Both the quantity and quality of protein in most sprouts are dramatically increased. New amino acids form as the seeds sprout, resulting in increased digestibility. In the sprouting process, the starches are converted to simple sugars, which rapidly enter the bloodstream when sprouts are consumed, thereby providing quick energy.

Costs vary, depending on the amount and type of seeds purchased, but even the most expensive sprouts would most likely cost no more than seven or eight cents per serving, making them very economical as well as a super nutritious food. Purchasing in larger quantities, would prove even more economical. If seeds are sprouted and regularly served, the food budget can be reduced without sacrificing the dietary quality or the health of your family.

Once the seeds have been soaked, rinsed, and sprouting has begun, they only require 10 to 15 minutes per day. There is no weeding, fertilizing, hoeing, watering, or working long hot hours bent over in the garden. You can grow them year-round in your home and do not have to worry about the weather or soil conditions.

Since sprouts are eaten fresh, you do not have to worry about preserving them, either by drying, freezing or canning. No packaging, labeling, transporting or storing is necessary. What could be easier?

Sprouts only take from 2 to 6 days to produce, and if grown on a continual basis, will supply your family with low-cost, fresh foods each and every day. Some seeds such as "quinoa," sprout in as little time as 12 hours. The nutritional support they provide is well worth the effort to grow them.

Seeds for sprouting can be obtained at your local health foods store or purchased on-line via the Internet. Make certain that the seeds you purchase have not been chemically treated in any way. Research your supplier! Purchase those sold for sprouting purposes only. Many times, seeds sold in seed and feed stores or nurseries, are chemically treated with insecticides to protect them from disease when planted in the soil.

Seeds must be stored in moisture-proof containers in a cool, dry place. Glass containers with tight-fitting lids work quite well. Date and label each jar and rotate them, always using the oldest first. Seeds cannot be stored indefinitely and still germinate successfully.

Purchase high quality seeds. Wash the seeds thoroughly and place them in a jar of 75 to 80 degree water and soak overnight in a dark location. Make sure to remove any broken, cracked or floating seeds, when you wash them.

Use plenty of water, as the seeds swell overnight and need to remain covered by the water. Save the water the following morning to water your house plants or use in any recipe requiring liquid. It contains essential vitamins and minerals. In the morning, rinse the sprouts and drain well. Always, rinse in cool water with a final rinse of filtered warm water, for quicker sprouting.

Place seeds in a proper sprouting container (I have found that sprouting seeds in a Mason jar hasn't worked well for me, I prefer an actual sprouting container). Follow instructions carefully for the type of seed you are sprouting and keep it in a warm, dark place such as a cupboard or closet. The temperature should range between 70 and 80 degrees. Rinse the sprouts with clear, filtered water and drain them well every four to six hours. If that isn't possible, rinse the sprouts in the morning, evening and again at bedtime. Let them stand for a few minutes in cool water when they are rinsed in the evening, allowing them to soak up the water if they haven't been rinsed every four hours throughout the day. Provide a final rinse of warm, filtered water and place them in a warm, dark place. Keep sprouts moist, but not wet. Seeds must not stand in water or they will sour and mold and need to be thrown away. Make sure that good air circulation is provided and that the seeds are not crowded. It may take some experimenting on your part to perfect the process, but will be well rewarded in the end!

Once sprouts have grown according to directions for that particular seed, it will be time to harvest. Empty sprouts into a pan of filtered, cold water. Handle carefully! The hulls of the seeds will float to the top and can be removed. Discard any hard seeds that didn't grow, as well as any soft or brown sprouts. When rinsed, place in a colander to drain for one hour. You may also spread them out on a clean, cotton towel to allow draining. Sprouts will keep much longer if excess water is removed.

Store sprouts loosely in a covered, glass container in the refrigerator. You can also place a clean, cotton cloth in the bottom of the container to absorb excess moisture. Do not use plastic bags. Plan to use the sprouts within two or three days, just in time for your next crop to be harvested. Sprouts are a powerhouse of nutrition and soon will become a healthy alternative that you will want to enjoy every day.

There are many methods and ways to grow sprouts. Visit your local library or bookstore to read the many well-published books on sprouting. Soon you will discover which method is right for you.

¤¤¤

Listed below are some of the seeds that may be used for sprouting. Experiment with many and decide which tastes are right for your family. All these seeds are nutritious and health building. For instance, wheatgrass sprouts and juice is the closest substance to hemoglobin known and is therefore a phenomenal blood purifier and liver detoxifier. They digest themselves, invigorating you while requiring no help from your body to process them.

- Adzuki Beans
- Alfalfa
- Almonds
- Barley
- Bean Group (Black, Kidney, Lima, Pinto, Red, White)
- Chia
- Clover (Red)
- Corn
- Cress
- Fenugreek
- Flax

- Garbanzo (Chickpea)
- Lentils
- Millet
- Mung Beans
- Mustard
- Oats
- Peas
- Pumpkin
- Radish
- Rice
- Rye
- Sesame
- Soybeans
- Sunflower
- Triticale
- Wheat
- Beets
- Broccoli
- Brussels Sprouts
- Cabbage
- Cauliflower
- Chard
- Endive
- Lettuce
- Turnips
- And many others!

¤¤¤

Experiment with the many recipes you will find in your sprouting book. You will be amazed at all the things you can do with sprouts. They even make delicious drinks!

Every home storage program or pantry should have a variety of these seeds stored. In case of a disaster when you are unable to obtain enzymes from fresh fruits and vegetables, sprouts could mean the difference between health and illness, or in some extreme cases, perhaps even between life and death.

> Note: There have been numerous accounts of food poisoning from store purchased sprouts.
> Another great reason for growing your own!

~

MOTIVATIONAL TIPS

When extremely ill, I was unable to tolerate sprouts. I was extremely careful in my preparation, however the small amounts of mold found in sprouts made it impossible for me to eat them without terrible reactions.

As my health improved I was able eat an abundance of them and enjoyed various sprouts on a daily basis. I became very good at hiding them in dishes, which allowed my son to also adapt to eating them. He was eating sprouts months before he ever realized it and was steadily becoming more healthy.

Be creative!

~

"Of all the medicine created out of the earth, food is the chief."

- Sir Robert McCarrison, M.D.

8

GRAINS & NON-GRAINS

Variety and Rotation

Whole grains and whole-grain products have been staple foods for thousands of years in most cultures. Today, they are used as a common source of carbohydrates and an inexpensive source of protein.

Grains

Barley - One of the world's most cultivated grains, barley, has been used as food in ancient Egypt as long ago as 6000 B.C. It was used as the basic unit of the Sumerian measuring system from 4000 to 2000 B.C., and was even the standard form of currency in Babylonia. Today, most of the barley crop in the United States is used in beer production or as animal feed. When barley is sprouted and then dried, it forms barley malt, which is used in beer, liquors, malted milk, and is added to many processed foods as a sweetener or flavoring. Pearl, or pearled barley is the most common form of barley, but it is not a whole grain. To make pearl barley, the whole grain is ground until the hull and germ are removed, along with most of the nutrients. For whole grain barley, look for hulled barley, which has only the inedible outer layers removed, or hulless barley, which is a different variety that does not require hulling. Hulled or hulless barley is a good source of fiber, niacin, thiamine, potassium, iron, phosphorus, and calcium. Barley flour is an excellent substitute for wheat flour in baked goods, as it has almost the same consistency as white wheat flour and a bland taste. Hulled barley is usually used for flour, so the nutrients of the whole grain are retained. Many people who are allergic to wheat are also allergic to barley, so use cautiously.

Kamut - Kamut™ is a registered trademark of Kamut International, Ltd., a new cereal grain, it is an ancient relative of modern durum wheat. Although the Kamut brand wheat is thousands of years old, it is a new addition to North American grain production. Each kernel is two to three times larger than the size of a wheat kernel, and has a wonderful, rich and almost buttery taste. Though related to durum wheat, studies have indicated that many wheat-sensitive individuals can tolerate this grain on a rotational basis. It has 30 percent more protein than common wheat varieties as well as more minerals. Kamut is higher in nutritional value than any other strain of wheat. It also contains higher levels of sixteen of the eighteen amino acids found in wheat and higher levels of all of the major fatty acids. It can be used for almost any purpose where you would use whole-grain wheat flour. Kamut is delicious cooked as a hot cereal!

Millet - Millet was a staple food in ancient India, Egypt, and China before rice gained in popularity. The ancient Chinese considered millet a sacred crop. It is still extensively cultivated in the Eastern hemisphere, particularly in regions with primitive agricultural practices and high population density, because of its ability to grow under adverse conditions. It has been said that Marco Polo wrote, that during the reign of the Great Kahn, millet was plentiful and was prepared as a gruel cooked in milk, rather than made into bread, which the Chinese had not yet developed. This grain has not shared this popularity in America. We traditionally use this grain for birdseed. It is a tiny, bright yellow, gluten-free seed, with a delicate and light flavor and is rich in iron, potassium, calcium, B vitamins, and protein. Many who do not tolerate other grains can eat millet without experiencing grain-like allergic reactions and is one of the most easily digested grains. The whole grain can be used any way that rice is used, in casseroles or puddings. Millet makes a great stuffing for cabbage, or green peppers, in making breads, hot cereals and wonderful casseroles. Dry roasting millet before cooking, enhances its flavor and helps to blend in the flavors of other combined foods. Puffed millet is available as a breakfast cereal at natural foods stores and resembles puffed rice in taste and texture. Millet flour can also be purchased at natural foods stores. It has a grainy texture much like cornmeal, and is good made into mock corn muffins. Like cornmeal, it is also useful for coating vegetables or meat for frying. Millet tends to be more alkaline than other grains, which is another great reason for its use. It is also used to make a delicious milk-like drink for those wishing to avoid dairy or nut milks.

Oats - An ancient grain, oats are thought to have been developed around 2500 B.C. in northern Africa, the Near East, and the temperate areas of Russia. The Roman Empire, throughout Europe and Britain, also utilized oats in their diets. In folk medicine, oats were used to treat nervous exhaustion and insomnia. A tea made from oats was thought to be useful in rheumatic conditions and to treat water retention. Oats are high in protein, calcium, iron, and phosphorus, and have a higher proportion of fat than other grains. Oat bran has been widely touted as being able to reduce cholesterol levels. Oats contain natural antioxidants, which help foods stay fresh longer. They are naturally sweet, so foods made with oats require fewer sweeteners. Oat groats are hulled whole kernels of the grain, which take a long time to cook. They are wonderful when slow cooked overnight in a crockpot in a mixture of water, apple juice and cinnamon. Oat groats can be found at natural foods stores. Steel-cut oats are groats that have been sliced into pieces with steel blades, and were traditionally used for oatmeal. They also take longer to cook. Rolled oats are groats that have been steamed and run through rollers to flatten them. Quick-cooking rolled oats are thinner because the groats have been cut into pieces before rolling. Rolled oats are less nutritious than oat groats or steel-cut oats, because of the cooking done during processing. Instant rolled oats are partly cooked groat pieces rolled even thinner than quick oats. Instant oats are cooked longer during processing, and usually have sugar and flavorings added, making them less nutritious and more expensive. Oat flour is not exposed to high temperatures during processing and thus retains most of the nutritional value of the whole grain. Oat flour is good tasting, very fine, and sticky. Since oats have more fat and sugars than other grains, oat flour gives dough a moist sweetness and makes good yeasted bread and excellent pancakes.

Rice - The origins of rice have been debated for many years, but the plant is of such antiquity that the precise time and place of its first development may never be known. Rice is the staple grain of half the world's population and is gluten-free. Brown rice is, nutritionally, far superior to white rice and has more taste, but takes longer to cook. When refined, rice loses two-thirds of its vitamins, two-thirds of its fiber, and half of its minerals. Along with all the nutrients being removed in the processing, the mold is removed also. About the only good thing white rice has over brown rice is that it is less moldy, which may be helpful information for those with severe mold allergies. Enriched white rice has some vitamins added, but the fiber and minerals have been removed. There are many varieties, including short, medium or long grain brown rice, sweet brown rice, Texmati, Calmati, as well as specialty rice varieties such as mahogany, royal and wehani, to name a few. You should avoid using polished rice, Minute Rice, and other highly processed rice products. Rice is susceptible to a variety of diseases and pests, and usually is treated heavily with pesticides and fungicides while growing. Strive to always purchase organically grown rice.

Rye - Rye is used abundantly in Scandinavia and Eastern Europe. It has nearly the same nutritional value as wheat, but a stronger, heartier flavor. Rye is very closely related to wheat and should be used cautiously if you are allergic to wheat. Rye flour contains gluten and can be used to make yeast bread. It makes a heavier loaf than wheat and has a bit stronger taste. Most rye flour sold commercially has wheat flour as an additional ingredient. Rye cereal and crackers are also common in our markets today, however they too usually contain wheat as an added ingredient.

Spelt - Also an ancient grain, spelt has been in use continuously in and around the European Alps since the Gothic and Renaissance ages of Europe. The grain's "nutty" flavor has long been a favorite in Europe, where it is known as "Farro" in Italy and, "Dinkle" in Germany. Spelt is a gluten-containing grain related to wheat and a member of the Grass Family. The nutrients in spelt dissolve quickly in liquid and become more readily available to the body with only a minimum of digestive work. Again, this grain can many times be tolerated more easily for those allergic to our more common wheat. Spelt is light golden brown, similar to whole wheat and has a high nutritional value with lots of natural fiber. It is significantly higher in protein than wheat and contains beneficial fats, carbohydrates, vitamins, trace elements, and minerals. It is rich in B vitamins and polyunsaturated fats and amino acids. Spelt flour handles and tastes more like modern wheat flour than Kamut and is lighter and dryer. Its texture falls somewhere between whole wheat and unbleached wheat flour.

Teff - Teff is an ancient grain with a minimum of gluten. For thousands of years the highland Ethiopians have used this grain to make delicious flat breads called Injera. This bread is a soft, porous, thin pancake, which has a sour taste and is a major food staple in Ethiopia. There are many varieties of teff, but only brown, ivory, and red are grown in the United States. The seeds are extremely tiny, needing 150 grains to equal one wheat kernel. Teff has a mild, slightly molasses-like flavor and blends well with other ingredients. It is a very nutritional grain containing iron, phosphorous, thiamine, calcium, potassium, copper, zinc, protein and soluble and insoluble fiber. Teff is available as a whole grain or as flour. Whole-grain teff is delicious used as a hot breakfast cereal with a natural sweetener and a milk substitute. Cooked teff can be used in puddings and pies, and also makes a good addition to soups, casseroles, and stews. Uncooked teff can be added to baked goods as a substitute for sesame seeds or nuts.

Triticale - Triticale doesn't have a history that spans thousands of years. It was developed more than a century ago by crossing wheat with rye in hopes of creating a food grain with good baking qualities. It has a larger kernel, or berry, than wheat, has a higher protein efficiency ratio than wheat, and a higher percentage of protein. Gluten strands do not form as in whole wheat batters, therefore, wheat flour must be mixed in with any triticale bread recipe to make high rising bread.

Wheat - Wheat was originally a wild grass and is the primary grain in the United States and Europe. In fact, wheat is grown on more acres in the United States than any other grain. There are three strains. 1) Hard, or winter wheat, is high in protein and gluten. It is preferred for bread baking. 2) Soft, or spring wheat, is lower in protein and gluten. It is the best choice for cakes and pastry making. 3) Durum wheat is highest in protein and gluten. It is used to make semolina, from which pasta is made. Bulgar is made from wheat kernels that have been steamed, dried, and crushed. Couscous is made from durum semolina. Natural foods stores carry both regular and whole-wheat couscous. Both kinds cook quickly and are good in salads, hot cereals, and North African dishes. Since this grain is the most widely used in the United States, many people who are allergic to grains are allergic to wheat.

Wild Rice - Wild Rice is technically not a grain, but an aquatic grass seed, originating in the Great Lakes region of the United States. Much of the wild rice sold today is cultivated but some is still harvested by Native Americans. The nose of the canoe parts the tall, slender stalks of grass which are then beaten to remove the seed. The wild rice kernels that fall back into the lake are already germinated and establish roots for the next crop. Wild rice is more nutritious than rice and other traditional grains. It is very thin and grain-like with a brown-black color. It has a strong flavor and is used mixed with other types of brown or white rice. Wild rice contains a high level of B vitamins, magnesium, zinc and protein. It is also rich in carbohydrates and low in fats. This food is fairly expensive, so you may want to use it for special occasions.

Non-Grains

Three of the foods listed here are considered "non-grains." Amaranth, buckwheat, and quinoa are designated as non-grains because, although they are prepared and act much like a grain in both whole-grain and flour form, they are not a part of the Grass Family.

Amaranth (Pigweed Family) - Hunters in both North and South America ate amaranth before agriculture became a way of life. A staple of the Aztec Indians, amaranth has a history of use in many religious ceremonies and as a gift in worshipping their gods. When Hernando Cortes conquered the Aztecs in 1521, he burned the vast fields of amaranth to destroy the culture's nutritional and religious foundation. Despite the destruction, amaranth continued to grow in the wild, and gained popularity in this country due to its nutritional value and versatility. Amaranth is gluten-free, making it tolerable by many people that are allergic to grains. The seeds are extremely small and vary in color from tan to black. The taste buds may need some time to adjust, as amaranth has a very unique taste. It has a high level of protein, amino acids and is rich in B vitamins and minerals. Amaranth flour and whole-grain amaranth can be found at natural foods stores. Used commercially as an ingredient in other foods, such as cereal flakes, cookies and cakes, amaranth flour is also delicious in muffins, pancakes, cookies, and any recipe that does not require gluten flour. Try purchasing some puffed amaranth at your local health foods store. It tastes delicious and is so good for you! Amaranth can also be popped. In parts of Mexico, popped amaranth is mixed with honey to make a popular confection called "alegria."

Buckwheat (Buckwheat Family) - Technically a fruit, buckwheat is a relative of rhubarb. It was originally cultivated in China, and then traveled to Europe, finding its way into the cuisine's of Finland, Austria, northern Italy, and France. Dutch immigrants introduced buckwheat in America, as early as the 1600s. Buckwheat is not related to wheat, however contains a gluten analog, which can affect some people with food allergies, so use it with caution at first. Buckwheat is an extremely hardy plant, usually grown without chemical pesticides. The flavor is quite strong and is often seen added with common wheat flour in pancake mixes. Roasted buckwheat groats, known as "kasha," are available in fine, medium, or coarse grind. Unroasted buckwheat is also available whole and as a cereal similar to cream of wheat. Most buckwheat flour sold commercially is made from whole-roasted buckwheat and has a very strong taste. It is used in pancakes, cookies, muffins and other recipes. It is best mixed with other flours because of its strong taste. This grain has plenty of protein and B vitamins and is rich in phosphorus, potassium, iron and calcium. I am sure you will find this grain a tasty alternative to traditional wheat.

Quinoa (Goosefoot Family) - (pronounced "KEEN-wah") means "mother" in the ancient Quechua language of the Inca Indians. A nutritionally superior grain that was once the staple food of the ancient Incas, quinoa is in the same botanical family with spinach, chard, and beets. Russian thistle, the common tumbleweed of the West, is also in the same family. This grain is now grown in North America in the high regions of California, Colorado, and western Canada. This food is sometimes referred to as a "supergrain." Quinoa is a gluten-free non-grain and has a wonderful flavor and can be used in various recipes for added nutrition. There are hundreds of varieties of quinoa, and it comes in many colors. The most common in the United States resembles a tiny version of millet. It is extremely high in protein, which makes it a favorite in many vegetarian diets. In fact, it has ten times as much absorbable iron as corn or wheat, contains essential amino acids, Vitamin E, Vitamin B, calcium, phosphorous and iron. It cooks quickly and makes a delicious hot cereal that works great as a main ingredient in cold vegetable salads.

¤¤¤

Sprouted multi-grain bread that is baked at home or a bakery is by far the most nutritious. The bread should not be consumed for at least a 24-hour period, allowing the yeast to rest and become inactive. Freshly baked yeasted breads, consumed straight from the oven, are not easily broken down and cause digestive problems. Bread should not be stored in plastic as this allows for mold to grow. The bread should be stored in an enclosed breadbox and eaten within a short period of time, after the 24-hour rest period. An even healthier alternative is to bake unleavened bread, using no yeast. This type of bread is much easier to assimilate.

Note: It is best to rotate grains in your diet, even if you are not allergic to them. You will be receiving better all around nutrition, will adapt to new tastes and recipes and learn to enjoy new foods. Most Americans consume only common wheat and corn (corn syrup is a cheap sweetener and is used in many processed foods) in their diets on a daily basis, making them the two grains causing allergies in most Americans.

Source: Portions of the historical information for the above grains and non-grains were derived from the very well written book, *The Complete Food Allergy Cookbook* by Marilyn Gioannini (see Bibliography).

~

MOTIVATIONAL TIPS

When I was very ill, I was unable to tolerate <u>any</u> grains. I experienced extreme digestive disturbances as well as joint and muscles aches, which left me barely able to walk. I also experienced a rapid and irregular heart rate and uncontrollable muscle twitching which prevented me from sleeping. My thought process was disoriented and I was in a state of confusion most of the time. Once my doctor diagnosed my allergies, and eliminated them from my diet, I began to improve. I now am able to eat a minimal amount of grains and try to rotate and vary them as much as possible.

I discovered many delicious recipes for these grains that I never knew existed. I challenge you to go exploring at your local health foods stores, and learn to use all these wonderful and nutritious whole foods.

~

"The ultimate measure of a man is not where he stands in moments of comfort, but where he stands in times of challenge and controversy."

- Martin Luther King, Jr.

9

ALLERGIES

Reactionary Force

Over 70 million Americans suffer from some form of allergy and the numbers are increasing each year. The American Academy of Allergy, Asthma and Immunology states that allergies are the sixth leading cause of chronic illness in the United States. Some allergies are seasonal, while others last year-round. Most allergies are inherited. The actual substances that we are allergic to are not inherited; however the food we eat, the air we breathe, the things we touch can all trigger an allergic reaction. In fact, many food allergies are traced directly to the multitude of poisons in what we eat and drink on a daily basis. Being exposed to allergens at certain times when the body's defenses are low or weak, such as after a viral infection or during pregnancy, may also contribute to the development of allergies.

Webster's Dictionary defines an allergy as an "exaggerated or pathological reaction to substances, or physical states that are without comparable effect on the average individual." The sad fact is that many people in the United States today are no longer average, due to our toxic environment. It further defines allergies as "an altered bodily reactivity to an antigen in response to a first exposure." Symptoms include sneezing, respiratory problems, itching, rashes, muscle twitching, rapid heart beat, digestive problems, brain fog and lethargy, to name the most prevalent. The allergen itself is the specific protein substance that causes the body to react negatively. The presence of this allergen in the body causes a series of chemical reactions in the immune system, which result in individual symptoms.

Our immune system helps to keep us healthy by producing disease-fighting antibodies, which are capable of destroying foreign substances like viruses and bacteria that cause disease. In people with allergies, these antibodies are over stimulated and react to normally harmless substances.

If you have allergies and are exposed to an allergen, your body's defenses are mobilized. An antibody called IgE (Immunoglobulin E), is summoned and sent throughout your bloodstream, releasing histamine from the body's mast cells. It is the reaction to this allergen and antibody "conflict" that causes the majority of allergic responses.

¤¤¤

Listed are several activities that can trigger an allergic reaction to IgE:

- **Ingestants**: substances that enter the body through the mouth. (Ingestants consist of foods, drugs and environmental toxins.)

- **Inhalants**: the allergen is breathed in through the nose or mouth. (Common inhalants consist of pollens, molds, animal secretions and house dust mites.)

- **Contact Allergies**: enter the body through the skin. (Contact allergens include powders, lotions, shampoos, soaps, metal jewelry, latex, etc.)

- **Other Factors**: cause allergy aggravation. (Changes in weather, humidity, and barometric pressure. Infections and second hand smoke may also contribute to and aggravate a particular allergy.)

Signs and Symptoms

There are a wide range of potential signs and symptoms of allergies that depend on several factors:

1) Type of allergy
2) Level of exposure
3) Individual reaction

Because these signs and symptoms may indicate the presence of disease rather than an allergy, your physician should investigate them.

Do not make the mistake of just assuming you have an allergy. Only a proper diagnosis from a qualified physician can tell for sure!

Listed is a sampling of symptoms you may experience in an allergic reaction:

- **Eyes**: Itching, redness, swelling and tearing may indicate allergic conjunctivitis. Chronic sinus inflammation may result in what is commonly known as "allergic shiners," dark circles that form under the eyes.

- **Nose**: Runny, itchy, stuffy nose and excessive sneezing are symptoms of an allergy often labeled as "hay fever." Due to the constant upward pressure from wiping the nose, a crease near the tip of the nose may be common. Children continuously push upward on their noses in an effort to relieve runny noses.

- **Digestive Tract**: Stomach cramps, bloating, vomiting and diarrhea are often the result of food allergies. Infants as well as adults can be affected. Many infants are labeled as having colic when in actuality they may be having an allergic reaction to dairy products.

- **Lungs**: Shortness of breath, wheezing and tightness of the chest are symptoms of asthma.

- **Skin**: Itchy rashes, welts, blotches or hives can appear after exposure to certain foods, medicines, household chemicals, plants, animals or insect stings.

- **Hyperactivity**: Many people especially children become hyperactive or lethargic when reacting to an allergen. Sadly, in many cases these children are put on mind altering drugs to keep them in balance.

- **Increased Heart Rate**: Take the test yourself. Check your resting heart rate. Eat something you suspect may give you an allergic reaction. Check your heart rate within ten to fifteen minutes. In many cases you will see that it has increased dramatically within minutes. See your doctor to discuss the probability of allergies to the suspected food.

- **Muscle Twitching and Aches**: These symptoms mirror arthritis closely. Stop eating or exposing yourself to a suspected allergen and see if the symptoms disappear. You may be surprised to find that you do not have arthritis at all.

Allergy Categories

- **Animals**: Approximately 18 percent of the American population is allergic to cats or dogs as well as other household pets and farm animals. The allergen most likely to trigger animal allergies is the flaking of dry skin called dander. The hair, fur or feathers of the animal are usually not the problem. Proteins secreted by oil glands in an animal's skin, as well as the proteins present in the saliva, cause allergic reactions in some people. Allergies to animals can take two or more years to develop and symptoms may not subside until months after ending contact with the animal. Many people do not realize they may be allergic to their pets.

- **Food**: Food allergies develop when there is an IgE antibody to a specific food. An allergic reaction can occur within a few minutes or as long as several hours after ingestion. Foods that are consumed daily often tend to be what causes allergic reactions (ex: wheat, sugar, milk, eggs, soy, peanuts, fish, shellfish and corn). Many people find relief from their allergies to food by rotating their diet on a weekly basis. Non-allergic food intolerance is more common than true food allergy.

- **Household**: Dust mites, tiny microscopic creatures that live in mattresses and pillows, as well as in over stuffed furniture, and stuffed toys are the cause of many allergic symptoms. The dust around your house may contain other allergens such as mold spores, pollen and animal dander. Other common irritants may include cleaning products, tobacco, and cosmetics.

- **Outdoor**: More than 40 million Americans suffer from allergic rhinitis, or "hay fever." Pollen that is produced by trees, grasses and weeds play a huge factor in this. Molds are parasitic, microscopic fungi with spores that float in the air like pollen. They are usually found in damp areas such as the basement, leaf piles, hay, and mulch or under mushrooms. Molds tend to move inside during the winter months and can be found in bathrooms, dark closets and under the kitchen sink.

Treatment

There are three main steps used in the treatment of allergies:

1) Avoid the specific allergen
2) Medication
3) Allergy shots or immunotherapy

Life Threatening – Anaphylactic Shock

Sometimes enough inflammatory chemicals are released to cause a reaction throughout the body, such as hives, decreased blood pressure, varying degrees of swelling, mental confusion or dizziness, shock or loss of consciousness. This severe type of reaction is called anaphylactic shock and affects the whole body (systemic). It is essential that the patient seek immediate medical attention. Peanuts, shellfish, drugs, and insect stings are the most common causes of anaphylactic shock.

The best treatment is avoidance of the known allergen. Unfortunately, this is not always possible. All persons with a known life-threatening allergy should carry an adrenaline kit and be knowledgeable in the use of this medication.

Taking the premeasured dose of adrenaline pushes the blood pressure back up to normal and reduces swelling, especially of the airways. After self-treatment, the person should be escorted to the nearest emergency medical treatment center as soon as possible.

¤¤¤

A toxic body = a compromised or overactive immune system = allergies.

~

MOTIVATIONAL TIPS

I became allergic to most foods and many environmental allergens due to an extremely toxic body. Special imported foods, derived from root vegetables, which I had never before consumed, became my day-to-day diet for an extended period of time. As my immune system improved I was able to reintroduce fruits and vegetables into my diet. I am now able to eat all fruits and vegetables; but only a very limited amount of grains. I rotate as many of my grains as possible, eating very small amounts.

If your immune system is compromised in any way, you may begin to react to more and more allergens. Examine how you feel after you have eaten or after you have been exposed to allergens such as dust, pollens, molds, and chemicals.

During my illness my body weight plummeted from 142 pounds to 89 pounds. I couldn't eat <u>anything</u> without getting violently sick, nor was I assimilating any of the nutrients which I did consume. No portion of my body was left unaffected. I experienced every symptom imaginable and felt like I was dying every day, all day.

When I finally located my doctor, I was so ill that discerning the factors that aggravated the allergies was a difficult process. I am now able to distinguish between problems due to foods, molds, chemicals, etc. At one point in my treatment, I needed daily injections of over twenty-two different antigens in an effort to desensitize my body to various allergens. Today, I take injections in rare instances.

I practice a very disciplined schedule each and every day. That protocol is the topic of this book. Without this discipline, I am confident that I would have lost my battle as well as my life.

If you suspect that you may be experiencing allergic reactions to foods or the environment, I recommend that you locate a doctor specializing in environmental medicine and allergies as soon as possible. Your doctor can diagnose and begin treatment immediately to assist in rebuilding your immune system and proceed with desensitizing your body to the known allergens.

~

"A wise man should consider that health is the greatest human blessing."
- Hippocrates

Your Thoughts

10

CHRONIC CANDIDIASIS

The 21st Century Killer

Candida Albicans is a form of yeast that is normally found in the lower bowel, the vagina and the skin. In healthy individuals, the presence of candida albicans is considered a normal part of the bowel flora; the community of organisms that live in the lower digestive tract.

An overgrowth in the gastrointestinal tract of the usually benign yeast (or fungus) candida albicans is now becoming recognized as a complex medical syndrome called chronic Candidiasis, or the Yeast Syndrome. Specifically, the overgrowth of candida is believed to cause a wide variety of symptoms in virtually every system of the body, including the gastrointestinal, endocrine, nervous, genitourinary, and immune systems.

Normally, candida albicans lives harmlessly in the inner warm crevices of the digestive tract, as well as in the vaginal tract of women. However, as this yeast overgrows when immune system mechanisms are depleted, or the intestinal tract is damaged, the body can absorb yeast cells and other toxins. As a result, there may be significant disruption of body processes resulting in the development of the Yeast Syndrome. "Feeling sick all over" characterizes this particular illness. Symptoms include fatigue, allergies, immune system malfunction, depression, chemical sensitivities, digestive disturbances, joint aches and pains.

The causes allowing for this condition to exist can be complex. Some of the major culprits include a high sugar diet, processed foods, and environmental poisons such as chemicals and heavy metals and over use of prescription antibiotics. These existing conditions may cause the immune system to become overloaded, depending on other factors in any individual.

The opportunity for infection in women is compounded further with pregnancy, through multiple pregnancies and the use of birth control pills. The female sex hormone, progesterone, which elevates in the last half of the menstrual cycle, increases susceptibility to yeast infection in women.

Prolonged antibiotic use is believed to be the most important factor in the development of chronic candidiasis. Antibiotics suppress the immune system and the normal intestinal bacteria that prevent yeast overgrowth, promoting the proliferation of candida.

We are all aware that antibiotics can save lives, but it is a well-known fact, even in the medical community, that antibiotics are seriously overused. Conditions such as acne, recurrent bladder infections, chronic ear infections, chronic sinusitis, chronic bronchitis, and nonbacterial sore throats can all be effectively treated with natural measures.

With the widespread use and abuse of antibiotics, we should also be aware of the dreaded "superbugs" that are resistant to currently available antibiotics. According to many experts, as well as the World Health Organization, we are coming dangerously close to arriving at a "postantibiotic era," in which many infectious diseases will once again become almost impossible to treat.

> Note: The current rush to use Cipro for anthrax is very worrisome, as it is in the class of antibiotics which are used as a last resort.

A weakened immune system may relinquish control, giving the candida an opportunity to proliferate and transform into a harmful fungus. Candidiasis can severely harm one's overall health status, making normal daily activities almost unbearable.

When Candidiasis (the fungal form of Candida) is present, it can break down the mucosal lining between the bloodstream and the gastrointestinal tract.

This breakdown may facilitate passage of harmful toxins and allergens into the bloodstream—some seventy-nine different toxic substances have been identified in the blood. Once in the bloodstream, these toxins are free to travel to all parts of the body, where they produce a host of adverse symptoms and further weaken the immune system.

¤¤¤

Listed below are some of the major symptoms associated with yeast overgrowth. Experiencing consistent, regular episodes of these symptoms coupled with a general feeling of ill health, may indicate yeast overgrowth is present within your body.

- Fatigued, listless, lethargic feeling
- Feeling of being "drained"
- Poor memory
- Feeling spacey – "brain fog"

- Depression
- Numbness, burning, or tingling
- Muscle aches
- Muscle weakness
- Pain/swelling of joints
- Abdominal pain/cramps
- Constipation
- Diarrhea
- Bloating
- Persistent vaginal itch/burning
- Impotence
- Loss of sexual desire
- Endometriosis
- Menstrual irregularities
- Spots in front of eyes
- Erratic vision
- Drowsiness
- Irritability
- Lack of coordination
- Inability to concentrate
- Frequent mood swings
- Headache
- Loss of balance
- Rashes
- Heartburn
- Belching/intestinal gas
- Mucus in stools
- Dry mouth
- Canker/cold sores
- Bad breath
- White coated tongue
- Nasal congestion/discharge
- Cough
- Wheezing or shortness of breath

- Frequent urinary urges
- Burning or tearing eyes
- Recurrent infections
- Ear pain
- Food cravings
- Insomnia
- Sore throat
- Environmental sensitivities

¤¤¤

Many of the new illnesses today have a predator looming in the background as an underlying cause. That cause may be chronic candidiasis. Please recognize the fact that candidiasis is just a symptom of a toxic body. Your job is to find a qualified doctor to help you discover what toxins are in your body and what measures need to be taken to rid your body of them.

Although this information can help, the best method for diagnosing chronic candidiasis is clinical evaluation by a *physician knowledgeable* about yeast related illness. The doctor will use your past medical history along with laboratory techniques, such as stool cultures and the measurement of antibody levels to candida or candida antigens in the blood to determine if you have a yeast overgrowth.

Once you have been diagnosed or if you even suspect candida, there are many measures you can take to help control this condition. The single, most important ingredient is diet. If the total protocol suggested in this book is implemented, your chances of overcoming this illness is almost certain.

A number of dietary factors appear to promote the overgrowth of candida, ultimately affecting the intestinal flora. The most important factors are high intakes of sugar, dairy products, and foods with a high content of yeast or mold, and food allergens. At this point, the body is battling a vicious cycle. The constant and almost uncontrollable cravings for high sugar, high carbohydrates, and foods containing yeast causes the yeast to grow, worsening cravings. The more of these foods we eat, the worse the symptoms become.

The friendly bacteria (intestinal flora) in your bowels have far-reaching effects you've probably never imagined. These hard-working organisms produce a variety of substances that can prevent cancerous tumors, inactivate viruses, produce natural antibodies and vitamins, and reduce cholesterol and more (see Life Changing Products). Once this bacterium is damaged by drug therapy, yeast can easily take a stronghold on our bodies and we can become very sick. The Yeast Syndrome can be found lurking behind many diseases in today's world. This is a very serious illness, which is being generally ignored today by traditional medicine and is further exacerbated by the use of prescription drugs to treat symptoms.

Along with my protocol, your doctor can assist in identifying a specialized regimen for you to follow that will assist you in detoxifying your body, rebuilding your immune system and maintaining your health.

~

MOTIVATIONAL TIPS

This section is very near and dear to my heart. In my search for a cure for my undiagnosed illness, I came to realize that I was experiencing approximately 98 percent of these symptoms. Upon further research, I realized that my son was also experiencing many of these symptoms.

We were both administered antibiotics frequently for recurring infections in the past. I was diagnosed with heavy metal and chemical poisoning as well. After realizing how toxic our bodies were and working with my doctor for an extended period of time, I now rarely experience these symptoms. We have had no antibiotic or other drug treatment in five years. Bronchitis, ear and bladder infections are rare and when they do flare up, I treat them with herbs, whole foods, saunas and other immune building practices. These treatments are effective without the dangerous side affects of antibiotics.

Discipline and commitment to a permanent lifestyle change is required to conquer chronic illness, granting you many years of vibrant health.

Much research has been done in this field and is available at your local bookstores as well as on the Internet. Take advantage of it (see Bibliography).

~

"One man with courage makes a majority."
- Andrew Jackson

Your Thoughts

11

PARASITES

Your Dinner Companions

A "parasite" is technically an organism that is receiving food and shelter at the expense of another organism, without giving anything in return. That host organism is you! The parasite lives a parallel life inside your body, feeding off your energy, your cells or the food you eat, reproducing rapidly. They are even feeding off the health supplements you take, considerably reducing the effectiveness of these compounds. Are you wasting your money on supplements? You must rid yourself of the parasites before you can begin to absorb your food or supplements.

Humans play host to over one hundred different kinds of parasites, ranging in size from microscopic, to tapeworms several feet long. The goal of a parasite is to remain undetected. In fact, the ability of a parasite to attain this goal is essential to its survival.

Research shows that from 85 to 95 percent of American adults has at least one form of parasite living in their bodies. Approximately one hundred different types of parasites exist today, which can be picked up anywhere you find bacteria, viruses or germs.

¤¤¤

Some common symptoms of parasites in humans are listed below:

- **Constipation**: Some worms can obstruct certain organs. Parasites can block the common bile duct and intestinal tract causing constipation. Constipation can also be caused by incorrect eating habits. The ingestion of white flour products, preservatives, sugars, and animal as well as artificial fats, may cause build up on the colon walls, which creates a perfect environment for hungry parasites.

- **Diarrhea**: Parasites can lead to frequent watery stools. Certain parasites produce a hormone-like substance found in various human tissues, which creates sodium and chloride loss that can lead to diarrhea.

- **Irritable Bowel Syndrome**: Parasites can irritate and coat the intestinal wall, leading to a variety of gastrointestinal symptoms and cause inadequate absorption of vital nutrients.

- **Aching Joints**: Parasites can migrate to encrust (become enclosed in a sac) in joint fluids. This is painful and is often assumed to be arthritis. Joint pains and inflammation are also the result of tissue damage caused by some parasites.

- **Anemia**: Some intestinal worms attach themselves to the mucosal lining of the intestines and rob vital nutrients from the human host. If they are present in large numbers, they can create enough blood loss to cause iron deficiency or pernicious anemia.

- **Allergies**: Parasites can irritate and perforate the intestinal lining, increasing bowel permeability to large undigested molecules. This can inflame body tissue, resulting in allergic reactions.

- **Skin Problems**: Intestinal worms can cause hives, acne, rashes, weeping eczema, and other skin problems. Cutaneous ulcers, swelling and sores, itchy dermatitis and many types of lesions can all result from parasite invasion.

- **Nervousness**: Parasite metabolic wastes and toxic substances can be irritants to the central nervous system. Restlessness, anxiety and mood swings can be symptoms of a systemic parasite infestation.

- **Insomnia**: Awakening during the night is possibly caused by the body's attempt to eliminate toxic wastes through the liver. Sleep disturbances can also be caused by nocturnal exits of parasites through the anus, creating discomfort and itching.

- **Fatigue**: Lack of energy, tiredness, flu-like complaints, apathy, and impaired concentration and memory problems can also be associated with parasitic infestation. The physical, mental and emotional symptoms can be caused, in many cases by parasites, which facilitate malnutrition resulting in improper absorption of proteins, carbohydrates, fats and especially Vitamins A and B-12.

- **Depressed Immune System**: Parasites cause this by decreasing the secretion of Immunoglobulin A. Their presence continuously stimulates the system response and over time can exhaust this vital defense, leaving the body open to bacterial and viral infections.

- **Excess Weight**: Dr. Donald Kelley, a leading expert in weight management, stated "Parasites are a major cause of obesity since they deprive the body of the proper nutrients and leave us only empty of calories and leftovers. The body also starts craving more and more food as it is starved for the ever-so-needed vitamins and minerals."

- **Other signs** of infestation can be excessive hunger, asthma, bad breath, diabetes, migraines, heart disease, and cancer.

¤¤¤

Parasites are a growing problem in the United States today. Our ever-increasing toxic bodies provide a perfect environment for parasites. Parasites thrive on the poor eating habits of humans.

According to Dr. Bernard Jensen, a foremost expert in colon research and therapy in the United States, "The average person over 40 has anywhere between 5 and 25 pounds of build-up in their colon. Parasites of all sizes thrive in this indisposed residue of fecal matter, slowly but surely toxifying the whole body."

It is important to eat foods that help cleanse the body of these organisms. Raw fruits and vegetables play a huge part in this detoxification process. A semi-annual herbal cleansing is one of the most important steps you can take to clean toxins and parasites from your body (see Life Changing Products).

It is equally important that you obtain high quality herbs, as well as herbs that specifically target the eradication of parasites. You can never truly appreciate total internal cleanliness and a sense of well being, until you have completed a program to clean your internal organs and intestinal tract.

Please note the following observations:

"I believe the single most undiagnosed health challenge in the history of the human race is parasites. I realize that is a pretty brave statement, but it is based on my 20 years of experience with more than 20,000 patients."
-Dr. Ross Anderson, N.D.

"We have a tremendous parasite problem right here in the U.S. It is just not being addressed."
- Dr. Peter Wina, Chief of the Patho-Biology, Walter Reed Army Institute of Research - 1991

"In terms of numbers there are more parasitic infections acquired in this country than in Africa."
- Dr. Frank Nova, Chief of the Laboratory for Parasitic Diseases of the National Institute of Health.

Note: Portions of the above information were obtained from the *Secrets of Robust Health Newsletter*, published by Secrets of Robust Health Publications.

~

MOTIVATIONAL TIPS

Parasites feed well from the human body. The smorgasbord before them is unlike any they could conceive. The fast-paced lives we live are conducive to happy parasites.

Our bodies should always be in a state of cleansing and rebuilding. Take steps today to begin an internal cleansing and begin to feel the difference in your overall health. Internal cleanliness is imperative to good health!

Research the evidence for yourself. Remember, herbs are powerful and should be used with caution. A qualified person, knowledgeable in the medicinal use of herbs should supervise your cleansing program. Please contact me for further information on natural cleansing centers.

~

"Truly, it is in the darkness that one finds the light, so when we are in sorrow then this light is nearest of all to us."
- Meister Eckhard

12

CHEMICAL EXPOSURES

Dying From Your Daily Dose

Our planet Earth is being polluted each and every day by all the chemicals we are pumping into our food, water, clothing, and atmosphere. It is well known that many of these chemicals cause a wide variety of illnesses such as cancer, birth defects, spontaneous miscarriages, lung disease, liver and kidney destruction, severe intestinal problems and irreparable neurological injury. Yet, only a fraction of the chemicals in common use today have undergone toxicological testing.

Chemical carcinogenesis is defined as the induction of neoplasms (cancerous growths), as a result of exposure to toxic substances. Chemicals with these traits may induce malignant tumors as well as benign tumors in humans or laboratory animals. Chemically induced cancer may develop many years after exposure to a toxic agent. An example would be the development of lung or bladder cancer, after years of smoking tobacco.

We regularly encounter a constant barrage of environmental chemicals, with 4 million distinct chemical compounds having been reported in scientific literature since 1965. Approximately 3,000 chemicals are deliberately added to food, and over 700 have been identified in drinking water. In addition, the number of pharmaceutical and recreational street drugs and the chemical exposure we face becomes overwhelming. Over 400 chemicals have been identified in human tissues, with at least 40 in breast milk, 73 in the liver and over 250 in blood plasma. The toxic chemicals are those such as chlorinated pesticides (DDT, DDE), halogenated, volatile and aromatic compounds, and organic hydrocarbons, fluorocarbons, and synthetic alcohols. Chemical agents in these categories include those such as trichloroethylene, benzene, chloroform, toluene, and xylene. There is also vinyl chloride, carbon monoxide, natural gas, sulfur dioxide, nitrous oxide, ethylene glycol, and synthetic ethanol. The list is enormous, but I assume you get the picture.

In many cases, disease is caused or contributed to by toxic exposures, involving low-level, long-term exposure that is not identified by the patient or healthcare practitioner. In such cases, the victim of the exposure is happily living his or her life unaware that slow poisoning is occurring. Such damage often results in, or contributes greatly to, a number of chronic and debilitating diseases.

Driving a car is probably a person's single most polluting daily activity. Nationwide, mobile sources are responsible for about 75 percent of carbon monoxide pollution. In urban areas, the motor vehicle contribution to carbon monoxide pollution can exceed 90 percent. Driving a car is a necessity for most of us; however, there are steps you can take to reduce your exposure. When driving in city traffic or on busy highways <u>always</u> use your "refresh" button. Never pull fresh air into the cabin of your vehicle.

Toxic chemical and environmental accidents are making the headlines regularly. However, for most of us, it is not the Love Canals or Chernobyl that directly injure our bodies. It is the constant, pervasive pollution of our air, water, soil and food supply. Just living, breathing, and eating in our modern world puts us at great risk. Much of our internal chemical intake now comes from indoor air pollution in our homes, schools, work places, department stores, and even our hospitals.

¤¤¤

Listed below are some of the most common sources of toxic exposure as stated in, *Optimum Wellness,* by Dr. Ralph Golan (see Bibliography).

- **Formaldehyde**: Plywood (especially that used for paneling), urea foam insulation, particleboard and pressboard cabinets, subflooring, furniture, fabric finishes, polyurethane foam rubber (used in pillows, cushions, mattresses and rug padding), mobile homes, fabric finishes, air deodorizers, some toothpastes, mouthwashes, germicidal soaps, some shampoos, nail polish and cosmetics, plastic food storage bags, insecticides, chemical fertilizers, smog, flame-resistant fabrics, televisions, waxes and polishes, adhesives, natural and synthetic clothes that are crease resistant, wrinkle resistant, water repellant, dyes, and moth proof wools.

- **Oil Vapors**: From oil furnaces, motor oil-impregnated air-conditioning filters, and electric kitchen appliances such as food processors, blenders, and can openers.

- **Combustion Products**: Carbon monoxide and nitrogen dioxide from gas ranges (especially in unvented kitchens), and from gas or oil heating. Kerosene heat is also extremely polluting.

- **Household Chemicals**: Dry cleaning chemicals in clothes, mothballs, rug-cleaning fluids, lighter fluids, the contents of most spray cans, solvents, paints, paint thinners, stain removers, varnishes, most detergents, scented soaps, cleansers (especially pine scented), air fresheners, toilet disinfectants, janitorial chemicals, ammonia, bleaches, window washing fluids, silver and brass polishes, furniture polish, tobacco smoke and petroleum based wax candles.

- **Herbicides**: Most all lawn and garden chemicals.

- **Pesticides**: Bug and fly sprays, residues on commercial food produce, residues from home exterminators, and cotton and wool clothing.

- **Ozone**: Electric kitchen appliances, such as refrigerators and freezers.

- **Fluorocarbons**: Teflon, spray cans, and Freon (which leaks from refrigerators and freezers).

- **Epoxy Adhesives**: On plastics and electronic equipment (televisions, microwave ovens, home computers, etc.), which releases gases when heated.

- **Automobile Fumes**: That enter homes and apartments from garages built under or attached to living quarters. Also when following vehicles on the highway with your windows open or your fresh air vent open.

- **Office Hazards**: Liquid paper, carbonless copy paper, ink, mimeographic and duplicating chemicals, copy machines, solvent based felt-tipped marking pens, and glue.

- **Chlorinated and Fluoridated Water**: Municipal tap water.

- **Polyethylene**: Plastic food containers, polyvinyls, (especially very soft and flexible plastics such as those in shower curtains, fake leather, and artificial flowers).

- **Polyesters**: Clothing, upholstery, drapery, furniture, sheets, stuffing for pillows, quilts, and stuffed toys.

- **Medications**: Those derived from by-products of petrochemicals.

¤¤¤

Removing exposure to toxic substances is an important part of holistic healing. A positive way to look at the gradual process of eliminating toxic and unhealthy things from your environment is that, at minimum, you will be significantly improving the long-term health prospects for you and your family. Beyond that, it is often found that removing exposures significantly improves health, eliminates symptoms and even some chronic diseases, which are often thought to have unknown causes. Why use unsafe chemicals for cleaners, deodorizers, pest control, etc., when there are so many natural, non-toxic alternatives?

~

MOTIVATIONAL TIPS

Commit to reading all labels on all purchases. Research the toxicity levels and facts behind the ingredients of each item. The information you learn will astonish you. Pass the information you learn on to others.

Americans are unknowingly dying a slow, deliberate death. Begin today and join the fight to minimize your exposure to these harmful and often, deadly chemicals. Your family will be healthier for the efforts you put forth.

~

"We must always change, renew, rejuvenate ourselves; otherwise we harden."

- Goethe

13

HEAVY METALS

How Weighted Down Are You?

Escaping contaminants from heavy metal poisoning is almost impossible in today's world. While the body is capable of adapting to its environment it has not learned how to dispose of heavy metals.

Human exposure to heavy metal has increased dramatically in the last forty-five years. Today, chronic exposure comes from lead in paint and tap water, mercury-amalgam dental fillings, residues in processed foods and personal care products. It is almost impossible to escape these toxins in today's environment. Most people do not associate chronic illness with the build up of heavy metals in the body. Symptoms can begin so mildly that you may not even realize you are not feeling well, and progress until you are finally diagnosed with one of the many names given to today's diseases. You are then administered prescription drugs in a futile attempt to assist you in dealing with the pain and sickness of the disease. The cycle continues. You become more toxic, take more drugs, become more toxic, until you either die a slow debilitating death, or decide to find out why you are so sick and begin taking steps to reverse the process.

The body tends to store metals in fatty tissue, the lymphatic system, circulatory systems, and vital organs such as the brain and the liver, where metals accumulate until a toxic limit is exceeded, affecting the functioning of the entire body. Particularly susceptible are people with weakened immune systems. Lead, cadmium, nickel, aluminum and mercury are the most prevalent sources of contamination. Over the years the FDA has banned many of the agents for contamination. The most noticeable bans include lead additives in gasoline and paint.

According to a study performed by Dr. R.M. Jaffe, Ph.D., the amount of lead introduced into our environment since the beginning of the Industrial Revolution is enormous. From 1720 to 1980, close to 55 million tons of lead were added to the industrial supply in the United States, and more than 7 million tons of lead has been used as gasoline additives in the United States alone. Much of this lead is now widely distributed on the earth's surface. For example, lead has been found at levels of up to 7,500mg per kg of house dust and the earth's crust measures at levels of only 15mg per kg. This means that urban soil and house dust can contain from 35 to 500 times the normal concentration of earth's lead. The sediment of United States lakes now contains about 20 times more lead than they did just 100 years ago.

Are you eating fish from these lakes?

While our state and federal representatives are concerned about the environment, as individuals we make personal choices everyday that can help us fight against metal poisoning.

A common symptom of toxicity is headache or a dull ache under the right rib cage, brought on by an overloaded liver. The liver must use its resources to detoxify everything before it can adequately take care of its numerous other tasks. Exposure to metals, chemicals, etc., tax the liver fairly quickly, paving the way for general decline in health as the normal functions of the liver are slowed (see Life Changing Products). For example, mercury in the nervous system interferes with energy production in individual cells, and the cell's ability to detoxify also becomes impaired. The cell then becomes toxic, and dies. Most chronic disease is not the failure of the immune system, but a conscious adaptation of the immune system to an otherwise lethal heavy metal or other toxic environment.

¤¤¤

Common Symptoms of Heavy Metal Toxicity

- Headaches
- High blood pressure
- Fatigue, weakness
- Muscle pain
- Joint pain
- Digestive problems
- Constipation
- Brain fog
- Hormone imbalance
- Depression
- Tremor, lack of coordination
- Hearing loss
- Liver and kidney disease
- Cancer

Sources of Lead

- Lead based paint and paint chips
- Solder
- Leaded glass
- Leaded gasoline
- Pottery glaze
- Newsprint
- Dyes
- Landfills
- Batteries (production and destruction)
- Inks
- Soil and air in and around industrialized areas
- Drinking water
- Sewage sludge
- Waste incineration
- Lead-soldered cans containing food
- Plumbing (lead-soldered pipes)

Sources of Mercury

- Silver amalgams (dental fillings)
- Paints
- Broken thermometers and barometers
- Fresh and saltwater fish and shellfish
- Grain/seed treated with mercury fungicides
- Fabric softeners
- Adhesives
- Mercurial diuretics/ointments/antiseptics
- Floor waxes and polishes
- Wood preservatives
- Cinnabar (Red Sulphide of mercury, used in jewelry)
- Some cosmetics
- Film

- Photo engraving
- Tattooing
- Plastics
- Histology labs
- Industrial wastes
- Air and water in and around industrial areas
- Sewage sludge and sewage disposal.

Sources of Aluminum

- Cans
- Foil
- White flour
- Some cheeses
- Buffered aspirin
- Deodorants (especially anti-perspirants)
- Tap water
- Food additives
- Antacids
- Sodium aluminum sulfate in baking powder
- Some infant formulas
- Aluminum cookware and cooking utensils

Sources of Cadmium

- Paints (artist's and commercial/industrial)
- Metals (metal plating)
- Colored plastics
- Fertilizers
- Fungicides
- Antiseptics
- Solder
- Batteries
- Gasoline
- Refined foods

- Fish and shellfish
- Coffee
- Meat (liver and kidneys)
- Poultry
- Grains
- Dairy products
- Cigarette smoke
- Landfills
- Sewage sludge
- Waste incineration
- Soil and air in and around cities and industrialized areas
- Car tires and soil along roadsides

Sources of Arsenic

- Insecticides
- Weed killers
- Ceramics
- Glass
- Paint
- Wallpaper
- Copper-smelting factories and soil from surrounding areas and downwind (sometimes for hundreds of miles).

Sources of Nickel

- Tobacco smoke
- Electronic devices
- Steel and metal alloys (jewelry, prosthetics)
- Air, water, and soil in and around industrial areas
- Hydrogenated oils

The above list was provided by Dr. Ralph Golan's, *Optimum Wellness Guide* (see Bibliography).

PRECAUTIONS

✓ Drink only purified water—and lots of it.

✓ Remove all dental amalgam fillings and replace with composite fillings.

✓ Change your cookware to enamel or glass. (Get rid of aluminum and yes, even stainless steel.)

✓ Use only natural cosmetics or cosmetics with your health in mind (see Life Changing Products).

✓ Stop using deodorant. Most of it is loaded with aluminum. Use apple cider vinegar. It will kill the bacteria that cause odor.

✓ Avoid antacids, generally, and specifically those containing aluminum.

✓ Do not smoke.

✓ Do not drink from aluminum cans.

✓ Eliminate metal dinnerware. (Use plastic, porcelain or wooden.)

✓ Stop eating shellfish. They are bottom feeders, where the contaminants are found.

✓ Fish, especially tuna, have comparatively high amounts of mercury.

✓ Many pharmaceuticals have heavy metals. Learn to use natural healing compounds from herbs.

✓ Remove all paints and cleaning products from your house. Don't even keep them in the cellar. Air rises!

✓ Don't eat food from cans. Can your own food in glass, eat fresh, dried or frozen.

✓ Certain types of occupations offer greater susceptibility to metal contamination. (For example: battery service workers, service station attendants, welders, dentists, jewelers and antique refinishers.) If applicable, protect your skin with long sleeved shirts and pants.

✓ Replace mercury thermometers with digital display thermometers.

✓ Take steps to detoxify your body on a regular basis.

TESTING FOR HEAVY METAL TOXICITY

Dr. Ralph Golan also states that, "Your doctor may not readily consider that your headaches, fatigue, recurrent depression, and abdominal cramps may be related to subtle heavy metal poisoning. But even if the doctor is willing to investigate this possibility, the standard tests measuring blood and urine levels of metals will not usually be accurate. Unless a person has accumulated an enormous quantity of these metals in the body, blood and urine levels may not be abnormal. These metals lodge in intracellular spaces (inside cells), rather than in the blood and urine, until very high amounts have accumulated in the body."

- **Provocative Chelation**: The standards set forth for testing heavy metal poisoning, by many of today's physicians, includes provocative chelation. A chelating agent such as intravenous EDTA (Ethylenediamine Tetraacetic Acid) or an oral agent such as DMSA (Dimercaptosuccinic Acid), extract metal out of the tissues into the blood and urine where it can be excreted. A 24-hour urine sample is then collected and tested for quantities of heavy metals. Chelation therapy with EDTA was first introduced into medicine in the United States in 1948 as a treatment for the lead poisoning of workers in a battery factory. Later the U.S. Navy advocated chelation for sailors who had absorbed lead while painting government ships. While undergoing this therapy, studies showed that the patients also experienced reductions in fatty plaque buildup on arterial walls as well as a reduction in hardening of the arteries. Thus, since 1952, IV EDTA chelation has been used to treat cardiovascular disease with amazing results.

- **Hair Analysis**: Another way screening can be done for heavy metal poisoning is through hair analysis. Hair is an easily accessible site of heavy metal deposits in the body. This type of testing can provide information on intracellular accumulation, as well the body's ability or inability to excrete metals. It aids in confirming suspicions of heavy metal toxicity long before abnormal levels show up in the blood or urine. Normal levels of toxic metals reflected by this test do not always correlate with the level of deposits in the tissues. This means that further investigation needs to be done. Testing of this nature should be done on hair that has not been colored or permed. If you have hair analysis, see that the laboratories conform to the standards set by the College of American Pathologists. Laboratories should participate in federally approved proficiency test programs as defined by the Clinical Laboratory Improvement Act.

¤¤¤

Once the metals are identified and the levels are known, several processes are useful in removing these toxins from the body.

Treatment is meant to perform three functions: 1) reduce or eliminate the source(s) of exposure, 2) reduce the body's burden of the metals with chelating agents, and 3) protect the body with antioxidants and other nutrients. As a first step, you will need to identify your sources of exposure and then to minimize or avoid them at all costs.

It is vitally important that you follow the protocol given to you by your health professional. It is also important for you to continue to research for yourself.

RESEARCH THE FACTS THEN……..REACT!

~

MOTIVATIONAL TIPS

Once an environmental physician was located that was able to help me, I set out on a journey to educate myself thoroughly on this subject. Doctors are busy and can't always take the time to tell you everything you need to know to protect yourself. Remember your health is <u>your</u> responsibility, not your doctor's. Traditional doctors also checked for metals through blood tests and most all tests were labeled "within normal ranges!" You must keep searching until you find the answer.

I changed my lifestyle completely and you can too! I do not use deodorant (an internally clean body doesn't smell bad). Daily saunas and showers will keep you smelling fresh and clean all day. I located a reputable company that uses safer chemicals and no heavy metals in their products. I use glass and enamel for cooking and use hard plastic dinnerware utensils to eat from. Do not put plastic dinnerware in extremely hot foods. The heat will release the chemical compounds which also cause toxicity. All wallpapers from my home as well as any old furniture with lead paint have been removed. I do not eat shellfish. I preserve my own food therefore reducing the necessity to purchase food in cans. I have also had many chelation treatments, detox regularly with herbs and take supplements daily to build my immune system.

~

"Make your own recovery the first priority in your life."

- Robin Norwood

Your Thoughts

14

AMALGAM FILLINGS

Poisoned With Every Bite

Mercury-amalgam dental fillings commonly referred to as "Silver" dental fillings, contain between 48 and 55 percent mercury. The American Dental Association originally denied that mercury from these fillings leaked vapor which is absorbed into the bodies of persons having this type of dental filling. Numerous studies to the contrary, have had to concede, that "silver fillings," do leak mercury vapor, one of the most toxic substances known to man. These fillings release mercury vapor into the body twenty-four-hours a day! Although more than a dozen new filling materials have been shown to be far superior to mercury-amalgam, it is still the most frequently used material in dentistry today.

Pam Floener, a spokesman for the Internal Academy of Oral Medicine and Toxicology stated, "The metallic mercury used by dentists to manufacture dental amalgam is shipped as a hazardous material to the dental office. When amalgams are removed, for whatever reason, they are treated as hazardous waste and are required to be disposed of in accordance with OSHA regulations and it is inconceivable that the mouth could be considered a safe storage container for this toxic material."

The chewing action that takes place with every meal wears down the fillings. Inevitably, we are slowly being poisoned with every mouthful of food we swallow.

¤¤¤

The symptoms displayed by mercury poisoning are vague at the onset. However over time the immune system is severely taxed and symptoms are numerous. Listed below is a sampling of some of the symptoms:

- Difficulty in concentration
- Easily agitated
- Physical exhaustion
- Inability to coordinate movements
- Headaches
- Muscle spasms
- Cold extremities
- Dizziness
- Blurry, irritated eyes
- Joint pain and stiffness
- Nervous heart (weak or rapid pulse)
- Insomnia
- Digestion problems
- Bleeding gums
- Sinus infections
- Metallic taste in mouth
- Frequent urination
- Numbness

As you can see the list is lengthy and the symptoms can be easily confused with other disorders. Mercury poisoning is rarely diagnosed and the symptoms are treated with drugs, further poisoning the body.

If you do have these fillings and decide to have them removed, it is imperative that you locate a dentist that is skilled in the removal and practices the precautions necessary to keep you from further harm during the removal. As fillings are removed the mercury vaporizes and is extremely toxic.

Listed below are eight steps that should be used in the removal of mercury fillings. The steps are presented by the IAOMT (International Academy of Oral Medicine and Toxicology). Ensure that your dentist is following these at a minimum.

1) **Keep fillings cool**: A removal must be done under cold water spray.

2) **Use of a high volume evacuator**: It is critical this be positioned within a half of an inch of the tooth at all times to evacuate vapor from the area of patient.

3) **Alternative air source**: All patients should be provided an alternative air source and should not breathe through their mouth throughout procedure.

4) **Air Purification**: High quality air purifiers able to remove mercury particles from the air should be running at all times within the room.

5) **Immediate disposal of mercury alloy**: Ensure that the particles of mercury alloy are washed and vacuumed away as soon as they are generated. The filling should be sectioned and removed in large pieces to reduce further exposure. Avoidance of grinding the filling into small pieces is crucial.

6) **Rinse mouth**: As soon as the removal has taken place the rubber dam (if used), should be removed and the patients' mouth should be rinsed for at least sixty seconds.

7) **Clean patient**: All protective covering should be removed from the room and patients face thoroughly washed. The doctor removing the filling should also take precautions to remove clothing and wash exposed skin as soon as possible, after extraction.

8) **Nutritional support**: A detox program should be provided to the patient. These nutrients should further aid in the flushing of mercury from the body. If patient has been diagnosed with mercury poisoning, chelation therapy (oral or intravenous), should be considered on an ongoing basis, until mercury levels are depleted.

¤¤¤

Once you have located a dentist that understands and recognizes the dangers of amalgam fillings sit down and discuss the procedures he plans to use in the removal. This is a vital step for your protection as well as the dental staff. You will also need to discuss what bio-compatible dental material will be used to replace the amalgam fillings.

~

MOTIVATIONAL TIPS

More and more dentists are seeing the effects of mercury poisoning in their own health. Take the time to research the facts surrounding this controversial issue. Locate a doctor understanding the dangers and who does adequate testing for mercury poisoning. Your next step is to locate a dentist who is qualified and understands the dangers of this toxin as well.

When inquiring of the possibility of mercury poisoning with my own health dilemma, most physicians and dentists told me that it would be rare this could have been causing my problems. It was not until I located a physician specializing in environmental medicine and a dentist who understands and practices safe dentistry, that proper testing was performed. Test results indicated I had extremely high levels of mercury as well as other heavy metals. Precautions were taken in the removal of all my amalgam fillings, replacing them with a less toxic resin material. I under went oral and intravenous chelation therapy for an extended period of time. I was also placed on supplements and foods that assisted in detoxifying and rebuilding my body.

Do not take this topic lightly. Research the evidence.

~

"Seize this very minute! Boldness has genius, power and magic in it."
- Jon Anster

Your Thoughts

15

ELECTROMAGNETIC FIELDS

Shocking Observations

The transmission of electrical energy through wires, the broadcasting of radio signals and the phenomenon of visible light are examples of EMR (Electromagnetic Radiation). EMR always consists of both an electrical field and a magnetic field, occurring in a wide range of frequencies. Cosmic radiation is at the high end; household electricity is at the low end. At this low end, is electromagnetic radiation referred to as EMF (Electromagnetic Fields). EMF is a broad term, which includes electric fields generated by charged particles; magnetic fields generated by charged particles in motion, and radiated fields such as television, radio, and microwaves. Electricity is the most common source of power throughout the world because it is easily generated and transmitted to where it is to be utilized. As electricity moves through wires and machines, it produces EMF. Once the electricity is delivered to our homes and offices, we, the human race, share occupancy with it.

In the workplace the generators of EMF include computers, cell phones, fax machines, copy machines, fluorescent lights, printers, scanners, telephone switching systems, electrical instruments, motors and any other types of electrical devices. Transportation methods such as automobiles, trucks, airplanes, electrical trains and subway systems are also significant sources of EMF. To compound the problem, more than one source of EMF in proximity to other sources will produce overlapping fields in the same area.

In our homes, the immediate sources of EMF include, electric blankets, electric water bed heaters, hair dryers, electric shavers, television sets, stereo systems, air conditioners, fluorescent lighting, electric can openers, answering machines, cell and portable phones, refrigerators, blenders, portable heaters, washing machines and clothes dryers, coffee makers, vacuum cleaners, toasters and microwaves.

While it is not completely understood what effects EMF have on human health, low level magnetic fields impact on biochemical and cellular functioning is well documented. The full extent of EMF effects will take more study. All research done on the serious health effects of manmade EMF has concluded that the adverse health responses from EMF are from long-term, cumulative exposure.

Certainly our forefathers were not exposed to the amount and duration of EMF that we are in this century. Since it appears that the adverse effects of EMF exposure increase slowly, over an extended period of time, we may never make the connection when diagnosed with leukemia, Alzheimer's or some other dreaded illness. Some scientists estimate that we are now daily exposed to 100 million times the EMF radiation of our grandparents. Research has shown that these fields have a significant disruptive effect on the natural energy levels in our bodies, triggering stress responses.

Both alternative and traditional doctors report that EMF is a co-factor in increasing our daily stress levels and the EMF problem has been categorized as a new form of pollution as serious as air and water pollution. Although our bodies are able to adapt to rapidly changing environments, the constant bombardment of man-made EMF can weaken our responses. Our immune system further depressed, sets up the perfect environment for disease.

Ponder this— Airlines require passengers to turn off their electronic devices during take off and landing, as it interferes with the plane's navigational systems. What do you think the effects may be on your own body's system?

In today's world it is virtually impossible to rid ourselves completely of EMF effects. We can, however, begin reducing the amounts of electrical appliances we use in our home and possibly even our offices. This may take some planning and sacrifices on our part, but I am sure you will agree our health is worth it. As small electrical appliances break, replace them with manual hand operated devices.

Since we spend one-third of our life in our bedroom, this should be the first room in the home upon which to concentrate. Remove as many electrical devices as possible from the room, one important item being the television. We truly only need one in the whole house and many would agree that we need none. Place fans, air conditioners, air cleaners, and lamps as far away from your bed as possible. Use a manual wind-up clock instead of a digital clock radio. Stop using electric blankets.

Learn to live without the microwave. Take the time to warm foods in small dishes on your conventional stove. Purchase a small appliance that can perform various jobs, such as a toaster oven that can bake and broil food, as well as toast your bagels. You can then eliminate your toaster, which can do only one task. Stop using electric razors and use hair dryers at a minimum, if at all. Cell phones and portable phones should be used only in emergency situations.

~

MOTIVATIONAL TIPS

These few tips should be just the beginning of your journey in your effort to eliminate additional sources of electricity in your home. Take an inventory of each room and set some short-term goals for ridding your whole house of unneeded appliances. Remember, the word is— "simplify."

Be an advocate at your office in cleaning up the environment. Work closely with your manager, making it a group effort involving co-workers. A healthier and safer workplace will mean higher productivity and less loss of time for company employees. Changing the lighting and adding screen protectors to computer monitors would be a good start. Moving copiers and faxes into an enclosed room would also be a big benefit.

Education and awareness is the key to this unknown villain.

~

"Setting an example is not the main means of influencing another, it is the only means."

- Albert Einstein

16

PERSPIRATION / SAUNA

Don't Sweat It - You'll Feel Great!

The skin is the body's largest organ of elimination. The surface layer of the skin, which is composed of cells, sweat pores, and sebaceous glands, is covered with a thin sheath of dead cells, which are continually being pushed up to the surface from below. If the dead cells are not removed, they can reduce and even block the skin's effort to breathe and eliminate waste, which is largely accomplished through perspiration.

Sweating is one of the most effective ways to remove fat-soluble toxins. Most of us do not do enough physical exercise in a given day to enable perspiration to remove harmful chemical toxins from our bodies; therefore, we must resort to other measures to enable us to sweat.

One way to encourage sweating is to take a hot bath with one half cup of ginger and one cup of Epsom salts added. (If you are pregnant or have high blood pressure, seek advice from your physician before using Epsom salts.) For a more soothing bath, you may add one cup of finely ground organic oatmeal. The water level must be as high as possible and as warm as you can comfortably tolerate. Drink a very warm cup of herbal tea or other heated, healthful beverage prior to the bath. Taking niacin helps to open capillaries however may cause flushing of the skin. This harmless, sunburn like symptom is temporary and is caused by histamine and heparin being released into the bloodstream. Cayenne pepper in capsule form, or taken in a bit of water will also encourage perspiration. Relax as long as possible; rubbing briskly every inch of your body twice with exfoliating gloves (see Chapter 19 for detailed directions for bathing). Rinse off with three hot showers, alternating with cold showers. Remember to work your tolerance up to the coldest shower possible.

Obviously the above method is the least expensive, but it is also the least effective method. My advice is to cut corners wherever possible and save enough to invest in a one-man portable sauna. We live in an ever-growing toxic world with chemicals invading our bodies through the air we breath, the foods we eat, the water we drink and bathe in, as well as all the cosmetics, deodorants, shampoos, and lotions that we apply to our skin. The only way to effectively remove these toxins is through perspiration.

If you are chemically sensitive it is most important that you purchase a sauna that is constructed without chemical adhesives and scented woods. Even if you are not chemically sensitive, it is better to not have this type of sauna. You can purchase a quality, environmentally safe sauna at a competitive price that is erected with untreated white popular wood and glass. The glass gives you a sense of openness, thus reducing the claustrophobic sensations that can be felt with enclosed wooden saunas. Stainless steel screws are used instead of adhesives (see Resource Guide).

Prior to doing a sauna, shower, using exfoliating gloves, to remove dead skin which will better prepare the body for easier perspiration (time may not always allow for this step).

Allow the sauna to warm for five to seven minutes. Start out with a lower temperature sauna of between 110 to 120 degrees for 30 minutes. As your body begins to perspire more easily and you adapt to the heat, increase the temperature up to 180 degrees for 35 minutes. Make sure you have permission from your doctor when taking saunas at this temperature. Take a large glass of water with you to drink while doing the sauna. Dry heat is more effective in allowing the pores to open and excrete toxins than steam heat is. It is also easier to tolerate dry heat. Take in a good book (none with glossy or new print), and relax. A bowl of ice water with a wet cloth may be used to keep your head and neck cool.

After your sauna, immediately begin bouncing on your mini-trampoline to continue the internal chelation process (see Chapter 22). Start out slowly and work up to a minimum of 1,000 jumps per day. After finishing on the trampoline, wait 10 minutes before showering. Your body continues to perspire for ten minutes after you stop exercising. Follow the process for showering in Chapter 19. When you step out of the shower, you will feel like *Tony the Tiger*, ready to take on the world. No matter how sick you are, this will make you feel better immediately. The best lubrication for the skin is organic extra virgin olive oil. Keep a bottle in the bathroom and smooth into damp skin. If a more intensive treatment is needed, a proven product backed by scientific research is "Formula III" (see Life Changing Products). In general, most lotions have harmful chemicals and should be avoided. This whole process shouldn't take more than one- and- one-half-hours.

It is very important that you drink lots of water after your sauna. You have lost vital minerals and nutrients as well as toxic chemicals while perspiring.

Saunas should be taken every day if you are very sick. However you must work closely with your physician ensuring you are not losing too many minerals. As you heal you can cut back to every other day and then twice a week.

Everyone should sauna at least twice a week.

It is important that you follow your physician's instructions regarding nutritional supplementation through this process. I personally take cleansing herbs for the colon prior to the sauna as well as 1000mg of Vitamin C. I also take non-flush niacin and cayenne pepper to enhance the perspiration.

If you do not have a personal sauna at home you may go to your local YMCA or exercise facililty. However, remember that these saunas are prone to mold and bacteria. You do not want to subject your immune system to any of these pathogens if at all possible.

A sauna is the single most important investment you can make for your ongoing health.

~

MOTIVATIONAL TIPS

I have completed over six hundred saunas and greatly attribute my renewed health to this entire process. When you are ill, your body will shut down the system it needs the least to direct energies to vital organs. I did not perspire for over two years. It took approximately five saunas for me to begin to perspire again. When I finish doing a sauna now, it looks like I have just stepped out of the shower. The euphoric sensation I feel when I complete this process each morning renews my confidence in believing my body can, in fact, heal itself if correct measures are taken.

I am so happy today, that I did not give up. However ill you may feel when arising each morning, make this process a part of your daily routine. Once you begin, it will become habit and you will not want to start your day without it. Your body will thank you!

~

"Come to the edge,' he said.
They said, "We are afraid."
Come to the edge,' he said.
They came.
He pushed them.
And they flew."
- Peter McWilliams

Your Thoughts

17

STRESS

The Untamed Killer

Most Americans have an enormous amount of stress in their daily lives. A large portion of the population hit the floor running when arising in the morning and are exhausted by the end of day. Stress is probably one of the most commonly used words in today's society, but is not new to the human condition. It has always been present, but is now more prevalent as the pressure and demands of this century take their toll. The word "stress" is derived from the Latin word *stringere,* which means "to draw tight." The modern word "uptight" accurately describes the response to stress.

Amid the hustle and bustle of modern everyday life, most of us keep going until we finally drop, usually late at night, from exhaustion. We are continually going full-speed ahead, living at a fast pace, borrowing on the store of energy we possess and robbing ourselves of needed rest to gain the maximum achievement and enjoyment in life.

Whether we admit it or not, stress is a number one killer, depleting our lives of vitality and health. It is believed that 80 percent of modern diseases have a stress-related background. Some of the symptoms of stress include; headaches, insomnia, muscle tension, digestive problems, and irritability. This is just a snapshot of the symptoms caused by stress. Stress is the catalyst of many illnesses plaguing our country. We fear diseases such as cancer, tuberculosis, leukemia, and heart disease and immediately think of treatment and medication, not necessarily the underlying cause.

When we hear the term "stress," we tend to dismiss it as if it were the common cold. The truth is that stress kills from the inside out. Whenever we experience fear or other feelings that create stress, our bodies release adrenaline which is secreted from the adrenal glands that lie on top of the kidneys. Adrenaline was designed to give the body that extra energy boost to escape from danger. Unfortunately, it can also make us feel anxious, nervous, and stressful.

There are multitudes of medications in today's market to help you deal with stress. Although they may be helpful in a temporary stressful situation, they can't remove the stress from your life. These medications also affect other aspects of the body. You must reduce stress by removing or adding "conditions or situations" in your life.

There are many programs, books, and self-help audio/video tapes on ways to reduce stress. While these tools can be useful in teaching us how to deal with stress, the best resolution is **reducing** stress in our lives.

The reduction of stress hinges on a single word - **SIMPLIFY!**

¤¤¤

You are the only person that can take steps to do this. There may be areas in your life that you can't simplify, but I would wager there are very few. Let's look at one of the biggest problem areas – **MONEY!**

- **Credit Cards** - Do not use them. If you do choose to use them, they should be utilized as a convenience only, paying them in full, with no interest, as soon as you receive your monthly billing statement. Unpaid bills cause many sleepless nights and much stress for people in America today. If you can't afford to pay cash, do not buy it.

- **Auto** - When purchasing your next vehicle, really assess what your needs are? Do you really need a new one? I bet not! How many times do you see a person driving a big, beautiful, loaded 4 x 4 extended cab truck without one speck of dirt on it? Most of these same people would never dream of hauling anything in that beauty, either. What is the true purpose of this vehicle? In all honesty, the answer is "It makes me feel good to drive it." Why do they feel good? Because other people are looking at them. Now is that a good reason to have a huge auto payment for five years? Do your homework and you can land a great used vehicle that will meet all your needs. The Internet provides some great sites to research automobile costs, dependability, safety, options and much more. You can determine the value of the car you wish to purchase as well as the value of the car you are currently driving. Purchase a car with as few extra options as possible. After all you only need to get from point A to point B and probably do not need most of the options. Talk to the previous owner to get the history of the car. Don't trade in your old car. Sell it yourself and save dollars. Refuse to pay sticker price! A great website to get all the information you will need is (www.edmunds.com).

Once you purchase your car, maintain it regularly. Don't become excessive with washes and waxes. Get a high quality, once-a-year car polish and polish it once a year only! Every time you are tempted to purchase the beauty on the showroom floor, remember you only need it for transportation, not appearances.

- **Clothing** - Be conservative. Select designs that do not go out of style in one season. Purchase coordinates whereby you can create several different outfits. Dry cleaning is extremely expensive and unsafe. Buy cotton, linen, wool, hemp or other natural fabrics. You do not need twenty different outfits or twenty different pairs of shoes. Buy only the basics!

- **Hair** - Get a cut that is easy to care for and doesn't need perms or colors. The chemicals are poison to the system and will damage your hair. They are also expensive and will take more time out of your already busy schedule to apply and maintain.

- **Accessories** - How much sterling silver or gold jewelry do you really need to wear? How many heavy perfume fragrances do you need sitting on your bedroom dresser? Do you really need a different purse for every outfit?

- **Home** - Get rid of the clutter! If you haven't used it within the last year, chances are you aren't going to use it at all. Have a garage sale and use the money to help others or take a much needed vacation. You will be glad you did! Do a complete and thorough house/garage cleaning twice a year and do the basics the remainder of the year. Our homes should reflect our minds and thoughts. If your home is clean, organized and simple, chances are your mind will be also. Your home should be just big enough for you to live in comfortably. After you throw out all the junk, you will see that you really don't need to move to a three-story Victorian home. The bigger the house, the more time you will spend in cleaning and maintenance.

- **Lawns** - Our lawns should be well manicured but not to the extreme. Instead of having perfectly spaced bulbs in a weedless garden, sow some wildflowers and give it the "forever wild" look. You will begin to notice the beauty in natural landscaping. Your neighbor will too. After all, isn't it the people that drive by our homes and lawns that we are actually seeking to impress? Be honest.

   The time spent outside would be better put to use if you were growing your own fruits and vegetables. This too can be hard work, but it is truly rewarding to know you preserved the food that will be served on your table throughout the winter months. You can take pride in the fact that your family's health is rated high on your priority list. Once the winter sets in, you truly will not care if your lawn was weed free and if the grass was kept at an exact height all summer.

- **Vacations** - Vacations are needed by everyone. However you don't have to spend thousands of dollars each year to take the whole family to a far away island. Your children will better remember and appreciate one or two vacations of this nature in their lifetime, than trying to sort out which island they went to in what year. A cabin or tent in the woods for a week or two in the summer will be equally rewarding. Children are satisfied spending quality time with their family and friends in their own backyard. Remember, the object of a vacation is rest and relaxation. Most people return more stressed and exhausted than when they left for vacation.

- **Extra Curricular Activities** - Activities of all kinds are fun and we should enjoy them. The key is moderation. How many parents rush home three to five nights a week, throw something on the table for dinner and spend the next three hours sitting at their children's ball game. They then rush home to wash the dishes with dried on food from dinner, wash the game uniform to be worn for tomorrow night's game, take a shower from sitting in 90 degree temperatures, feed the dog, assist with homework, lay clothes out for the next day, pack lunches for tomorrow, or worse yet, throw the child a dollar to purchase a non-nutritious, fat-sugar-salt filled lunch at school. That description was exhausting and so are we after doing all that. The list is never ending, but I think you get the picture. When you have several children participating in sports, it gets unmanageable. Each season brings with it a new sport or activity. We never stop running. Our children should have the opportunity to try several different sports or activities. Allow them to choose one or two they truly enjoy and concentrate on them for that year. Is running to games, dance classes, etc. (every night) true quality time spent with your family? Think long and hard about this one. Extra curricular activities after school and after work are one of the most stressful things we do to our children and ourselves. What are we teaching our children? Will they grow up more stressed than we are? What are we doing to our health? Our lives?

- **Toys** - We all love them and manage to save money or take out loans to get them - cars, boats, motorcycles, ATV's, snowmobiles, and jet skis. Most of us have certain hobbies such as train collecting, antiques, trips to the racetrack or the casino, nights out with the boys/girls, etc. I am not advocating that we shouldn't strive to do or get things we enjoy. What I am saying is that each of us should evaluate the trade off. We all need some form of recreation, but are the costs of these toys and activities bringing more stress into our life than pleasure? Are we working at an all-consuming job to pay for them leaving no time for enjoyment? You must make your own determination.

- **Careers** - All of the above issues will ultimately decide what career you will choose. It seems most Americans are not doing in life what they would choose. Money and recognition is the driving force in our careers today. We make more money, we spend more money. We get recognized, we want more recognition. We strive to climb higher. That is a sad fact! We are not content where we are. Most professionals are trying at all costs to climb the ladder of success. What is success? Is it earning a six-figure income? Is it traveling all over the world on business? Is it shaking hands with the most elite? I challenge you to ask some retired professional men and women who have had these opportunities. In most cases, their response is "I wished I had spent more time with my family and doing those things I enjoy most." If they had it to do over again they would approach life differently. Shouldn't we take this tried and proven advice for ourselves, before it is too late and we are chanting the same words they are? This constant driving force is affecting our physical and mental health. We are stressed to the point that by the time we retire, we keel over from a heart attack or need to take radiation and chemotherapy treatments on a weekly basis, grasping for a few more years. Our families are being torn apart. Juvenile crime and corruption is escalating. When the family unit is broken and single parents are bringing up the children, it is a fact that they will be adversely affected. Dads can't be Moms and Moms can't be Dads. The true functional family needs both. I don't care how many reports you read that tell you differently. We supply our children with all the material possessions they can possibly dream of, but try as we might; we do not supply them with quality time, devotion or true parental love in many cases. Spouses spend more time at work with their co-workers than they do with each other. Is it any wonder that divorce rates are so high?

- **24-Hours of Rest** - Each of us, including our children need a complete day of rest, removing ourselves from the activities that make up the other six days of the week. This doesn't mean you have to lie on the sofa all day but it may mean taking a nap in the afternoon. We need to rest in terms of our minds as well as our bodies. Resting can mean worshipping our creator and being thankful for all we have been given. Walking in nature with our children is a wonderful form of rest and relaxation. Helping others is actually a form of rest. When we reach out to meet another person's needs, our bodies actually respond in a healing and rejuvenating manner. This doesn't mean you should mow your neighbor's lawn all day and he mows yours, but it could mean visiting a nursing home or extended care facility with your family on the day of rest each week. Visiting someone (even a total stranger) who may not have family that comes to visit is a wonderful experience for you and your children. Bring a bud vase of flowers or other small gift. This will teach your children to give not only of their time, but also of the money they may have earned.

- **Seek Out Neighbors** that may be suffering in some way. Once you find these people you will have ideas galore as to ways you can bring joy to their lives. Sometimes it may be financial, other times it may be just time spent with them in conversation. Most people in America today are very lonely. That's right, even those of us who are busy 24-hours a day. Once you have experienced this type of rest, your stress level will be drastically reduced. You will begin to realize the important things in life and what really matters.

Is it time that you gave up some of your material possessions and take on a job that will allow you to spend more time with your family? Before you leave this section of the book, take time to evaluate your life as it is today. Spend the next month thinking of ways you can simplify your life, allowing you to exist on less. You have only one chance at life here on planet Earth. We all want to live long, healthy lives, but it doesn't "just" happen. We have to plan and work at it.

~

MOTIVATIONAL TIPS

Gather your family together this week to discuss what steps you can take that will enable you to rest from normal day-to-day activities. Set aside one day each week for rest and relaxation. Saturday, the Sabbath of our Lord is the day He chose for us to rest.

When we serve others, something magical happens. Our lives are more fulfilled; we are happier, healthier and end up with more time available to us than if we hadn't reached out. Try it. It works!

Another important step is to make a list of outstanding debts. Make a decision today that you are going to reduce your debts in a reasonable manner (not by working another fifteen hours per week). Employ the assistance of a professional, to help you if needed. You may possibly consolidate or need to part with some of your toys. Whatever the steps that are required of you to reduce your debts, they will, in some way come back to you as a blessing.

Last, but certainly not least, let go of past hurts, anger and resentment for any other person. The negative and harmful feelings only harm you, not the other person. Your immune system is constantly being lowered by these feelings. Surround yourself with positive and upbeat people. Before you know it, you will be content in your current situation. You will be setting new goals with reasonable expectations. This new change in you will bring with it new priorities, new opportunities and renewed hope. Tried, true and thrilling facts!

~

"A good rest is half the work."
- *Yugoslav Proverb*

18

BREATHING

Waiting To Exhale

Did you ever stop to think that we live at the bottom of an ocean of air that surrounds the globe? We could live a few weeks without food and a few days without water. However, if the ocean of air were to disappear we would all be unconscious within one or two minutes and within five or six minutes we would be dead.

Oxygen is the single most important element we take into our body. We need a constant supply of pure air into our bodies to keep our blood pure, to soothe our nervous system and to expand and keep our lungs healthy. Without oxygen, life would cease to exist. The lungs capture oxygen, which in turn provides energy, and then release carbon dioxide, which is the "exhaust" from cells. Oxygen is exchanged for carbon dioxide in tiny sacs called "alveoli." In order for this exchange to take place efficiently, good circulation within the lungs is essential.

Although most people realize the importance of oxygen many people do not know or use proper breathing techniques, which will maximize the effect of every breath.

Your body is most toxic after you have slept all night and have done shallow breathing for eight hours or more. Upon waking each morning, immediately step outside into the fresh air and take deep breaths until you feel lightheaded. Stand with your head erect, holding your shoulders back and pushing your chest out. Place your hands on your back rib cage just above the waist, fingers spread apart and pointing towards your spine. This enables you to make sure your lungs are expanding at the bottom, and prevents the customary shallow breathing at the top of the lungs. When doing this exercise properly the shoulders should not move up and down, but the rib cage should move in and out. Inhale slowly through the nose, expanding the chest gradually until your lungs can hold no more. Hold to the count of ten, and exhale slowly through the mouth, deflating your lungs completely. Inhaling through your nose is most important, as it collects pollens, dust, molds and other allergens, preventing them from being inhaled into the lung cavity.

To maximize the lungs' potential and efficiently utilize the oxygen taken in, you need to be aware of your breathing patterns. With a few exceptions, you should always breathe deeply, continuously clearing toxins from your lungs. As this concept becomes embedded into your mind you will consciously make yourself aware of the steps in proper breathing. A wonderfully euphoric state of mind will be present as you breathe deeply, strengthening your lungs and building your immune system. Increasing your lung capacity will greatly increase your resistance to coughs, colds and infections.

Long, slow breathing makes your body alkaline (which is good), while breathing rapid and shallow makes your body acidic (which is bad). Breathing a slow deep breath gives cells plenty of oxygen. Practice is needed to train the body to incorporate proper breathing techniques.

Negative ions, which are found in pure, fresh air, are invigorating to the body, causing the blood to circulate throughout the system. The negative ions relieve tension, calm the mind and promote an overall sense of well being. Proper breathing invites a wonderful night of sound, restful sleep.

As you master the art of proper breathing the next step in the process is to visualize your cells being renewed by the intake of pure, fresh air. As you exhale toxins that have been stored in your body, imagine releasing negative thoughts with each breath. Release feelings of anger, jealousy, fear, and doubt. Meditation and spirituality is further discussed in Chapter 27 of this book.

> **Note:** Negative ions make you feel positive, while positive ions (found in ill-ventilated areas) make you feel negative.

~

MOTIVATIONAL TIPS

Before going outside to do your breathing in the morning, jot down your feelings. After performing deep breathing exercises, record your immediate reaction. What changes have you noticed?

Periodically, throughout the day, ask yourself, "Am I breathing correctly?" Soon, it will become a habit and you will breathe correctly without thinking about it.

Be continually aware of your environment, striving for an intake of pure, fresh air on a consistent basis.

~

"Live life to the fullest. You have to color outside the lines once in a while to make your life a masterpiece. Laugh everyday, keep growing, keep dreaming, keep following your heart. The important thing is not to stop questioning."
- Albert Einstein

19

WATER

Let It Flow

All life is dependent on water. The human body is composed of approximately 74 percent water and is utilized by virtually all bodily functions, including digestion, absorption, circulation, and excretion. Water also delivers nutrients throughout the body, assists in maintaining body temperature and waste elimination. Therefore, replacing the water that is continually lost through daily sweat and elimination is very important. All chemical processes, by which the body functions, require an adequate supply of pure water.

Industrial and agricultural pollutants, which contain various toxins and carcinogens, have tainted our drinking water. When your water supply is contaminated and you drink it, the toxic chemicals are readily absorbed into the bone marrow, fat and internal organs.

¤¤¤

Common Water Pollutants

- Organic chemicals
- Inorganic chemicals
- Physical agents
- Biological agents

Organic chemicals are primarily from industrial and agricultural origin and include herbicides and pesticides. Water pollution is a continuing and widespread problem, leading to a multi-million dollar business in bottled water sales.

Heavy metals and chemicals are considered inorganic contaminants, which enter the water supply through industrial pollution, erosion of water pipes and leaching of acid rain. Much of the toxicity in our water at home is brought through the pipes; many of which contain lead and cadmium from solder and/or pipes. PVC pipes are made of petroleum that can leach chemicals when hot water runs through them.

Never drink or cook from water drawn from the hot water tap! Sediment stored in your hot water tank can be toxic, thereby polluting the water held in the tank. Always allow your cold water to run a few minutes to flush out stale standing water that may be contaminated in your pipes.

Chlorine and fluoride are commonly added to public water supplies. The benefits of these two chemicals are well known in the prevention of tooth decay. However there is well-documented evidence that these chemicals may exhibit carcinogenic traits and have been proven to cause bladder cancer in laboratory rats. Side effects from fluoride and chlorine include discoloration in the teeth as well as brittle teeth that are more prone to fracture.

While these compounds do kill some microorganisms, many viruses are not destroyed. Rather, these compounds do destroy beneficial bacteria in our intestinal tract which over a period of time, leads to digestion problems, constipation and diarrhea, disallowing our body the ability to assimilate food.

A point to remember. Chlorine is readily absorbed into your skin and vapors are inhaled through the shower. You must filter the water you bathe in as well as your drinking water. Taking one, 5-minute shower is equivalent to drinking four, 8-ounce glasses of chlorinated water, as far as the absorption of chlorine is concerned.

Physical agents are sediment of all types, as well as asbestos.

Biological agents are bacteria, viruses, parasites and fungi, all which are becoming more prevalent in water supplies.

Purification Methods

Carbon Filters- This type of filter helps remove organic compounds while allowing healthy minerals to flow. These filters may improve the taste and smell of water. Unfortunately, the filters will not destroy inorganic agents. Filters must be changed often or they will become a breeding ground for bacteria. If you have a whole-house carbon filter and a good degree of iron bacteria in your water (which many homes do), you may need a weekly filter change.

Distillation- This process heats the water to steam, and then recondenses to water, freeing water of the inorganics and physical impurities. The final product must be distilled at least three times to be free of organic materials. The process of distillation removes all healthful minerals from the water. It becomes very thirsty water when consumed and upon elimination, leaches beneficial minerals from the body. This method is fairly expensive and requires a good deal of maintenance. Controversy exists in determining if distilled or spring water should be consumed. Research the facts, then make an informed decision about the best water choice for you.

Reverse Osmosis- This method forces water through a semi-permeable membrane that allows molecules of water and healthful minerals to pass through unscathed. Most inorganic chemicals, organic compounds, physical agents, bacteria and other larger microorganisms are eliminated. Unlike distillation and carbon filtration, this technology doesn't actually trap or accumulate impurities. It is relatively maintenance free. If used with the carbon filtration system, the end result is tasty, clean water with some of its natural minerals. Although initial costs may be substantial for the combination system, it is inexpensive health insurance and one of the least expensive systems to maintain.

Some families opt to have spring or artesian water delivered to their home. If you choose this method be sure to research the integrity of the company from which you are purchasing the water. Plastic bottles may leach chemicals into the water especially when exposed to heat.

Drink water from glass bottles only!

You may also have your water tested at a reasonable price. You can send a sample of your water to be tested for heavy metals and chemicals as well as certain minerals. Just remember the problem may not be in the actual water itself, but may be in the pipes delivering it to your home. Follow directions exactly when pulling samples for your test and research the company that will be performing the water test.

There is an ongoing controversy concerning the benefits of soft water versus hard water. Hard water contains the minerals calcium and magnesium, which prevent soap from lathering and deposit a sediment film on hair, clothing, pipes, dishes and wash tubs. Although hard water can be annoying, studies show that deaths from heart disease are lower in areas where the drinking water is hard. However, it is believed by some that calcium found in hard water is not good for the heart, arteries, or bones. Unfortunately, hard water deposits its calcium and other minerals on the **outside** of these organs while it is the calcium found **within** these organs that is beneficial to the body.

Two types of "soft" water exist. One is natural, the other is manmade. Water is made "soft" by utilizing a treatment of sodium, which helps remove calcium and magnesium. Repercussions to manmade "soft" water include the possibility of dissolving linings in pipes. Lead, plastic, galvanized, and copper are all types of material used for the transportation of water. All of these have the potential of allowing harmful ingredients such as lead, cadmium, copper, zinc, and arsenic into the body. Research the facts for yourself and choose the water and water filtration system best for your household.

Now that you have some facts on various filtration systems, let's discuss the importance of water internally and externally to the body.

Internally

Water is a wonderful cleanser and should be consumed throughout the day. While water helps to give you energy, it also keeps every organ in your body lubricated and running smoothly. Water should be consumed at room temperature as extremely hot or cold is a shock to the digestive system and should always be avoided.

- Upon waking, a tall glass of pure warm water with a twist of fresh lemon should be consumed. Wait thirty to sixty minutes before eating any food. This is the most important water of the day. Your body is most toxic upon rising in the morning and this water will start flushing the toxins immediately.

- Never drink any beverage when eating. The stomach acids mistake liquids as digestive enzymes found in your saliva and will greatly inhibit the digestive process. Dilution of hydrochloric acid interferes with digestion and over a long period of time, causes an over production of hydrochloric acid and consequently, indigestion and acid reflux.

- Never gulp your water. Your stomach is not meant to be a holding tank for large volumes of water at one time. Water should be consumed in small amounts throughout the day. You should be consuming at least ten 8-ounce glasses of water per day or more. Water should become our beverage of choice.

- Do not drink any liquid for at least two hours after you have consumed food.

- Drink pure water from glass containers, not from metal or plastic containers.

- Stop drinking at least two hours before bedtime. Your bladder needs time to empty completely, enabling you an undisturbed and peaceful sleep.

Externally

Water is equally important to the external shell of the body. Daily bathing removes dead skin and encourages new healthy skin to grow. Removing the dead layers of skin opens the pores, enabling impurities to be easily excreted, thus aiding all internal organs in their work. The way you shower is equally important to your overall health.

- Each day, showers utilizing purified water should be taken. After exercising, a hot shower should be taken using exfoliating gloves. Once you begin using exfoliating gloves, wash cloths will be a thing of the past. Your skin will take on a new, healthy glow and be baby soft. Use a non-toxic soap (see Life Changing Products), rubbing briskly over every inch of your body **twice** with the gloves. Allowing the water to cover your head first, immediately rinse with cold water.

You must rinse your head first when changing water temperatures.

Sudden temperature changes such as cold water hitting the center of the body first, can cause blood to flow from the head too rapidly, giving a feeling of lightheadedness. If you have a heart condition, please check with your doctor before performing the hot/cold showers.

- The hot/cold water should be repeated three times with each shower. When you step out of the shower, you will feel absolutely exhilirated and energized. Once you get into the habit, no other kind of shower will be satisfying to you. The purpose of the hot water is to bring toxins to the surface for elimination. When the warm blood feels the cold water it will rush to internal organs in the center of your body to keep warm. As the hot water is once again applied, blood will rush to the outer surface of the skin bringing with it toxins accumulated from the center of the body to be excreted via the skin. Once the cold water is applied again, the process is repeated.

¤¤¤

Water is a very precious commodity and we can not live without it. It serves as a purification process both internally and externally.

Obtaining and consuming pure water is a number one priority in regaining your health.

~

MOTIVATIONAL TIPS

Prior to my illness, I never enjoyed drinking water. On the rare occasions I did drink water; it was chlorinated coming from a drinking fountain at school or work. I now drink from 2 to 3 quarts per day. During my recovery process I drank a minimum of one gallon per day.

Drinking lots of water must become a habit. Once a habit, you will consume it without thought and will want a supply of pure fresh water with you at all times.

~

"Eliminate something superfluous from your life. Break a habit. Do something that makes you feel insecure."
- Piero Ferrucci

Your Thoughts

20

SUNSHINE

Radiant Beams In Moderation

Did you ever stop to think that without sunlight there would be no life on this earth? Not a leaf could grow, nor a flower bloom. No animal life could exist and there would be no fish in the sea. It is from the tremendous power and energy given off by the sun that all life, vegetable and animal, receives directly or indirectly, the power to live and grow.

A secret to great health is utilizing as many aspects of nature as possible. Introducing products of nature ensures adding wonderful elements to our bodies without the risk of destroying body parts. The addition of vitamins and minerals by utilizing nature's inherent goodness, is a major part of having a healthy body.

One of the most natural ways of receiving Vitamin D is from sunshine. Our bodies do not produce Vitamin D on their own. Sitting in the sunrays will allow us to absorb ultraviolet rays, which will aid in changing serum cholesterol to Vitamin D within our bodies. Sunlight has also been thought to aid in increasing testosterone levels, lowering blood pressure, and treating psoriasis, tuberculosis, and neonatal jaundice. It is also instrumental in the treatment of SAD (Seasonal Affective Disorder). Vitamin D can be received via other methods including foods such as fish, egg yolks, and fortified milk, which in today's toxic world may not be the best foods to eat. Although foods exist that contain Vitamin D, nothing will replace the benefits of a daily dose of sunshine.

Sunlight effectively kills germs in the air, purifies water, destroys bacteria on exposed surfaces, and produces antibacterial agents on the skin from the oils that have been deposited.

The use of animal and refined fats in the diet causes complications. The fats are deposited in various places in the body, one being the skin cells. When sunrays strike these cells, those fats become rancid, causing the formation of free radicals. This causes damage within the cell structures, increasing susceptibility to sunburn, age spots, and greatly promoting not only skin cancer, but breast and colon cancer as well.

Many of the fats in sunscreen lotions deposited on the skin may also stimulate formation of cancerous cells.

It is essential to realize that direct sunlight in great amounts can be very dangerous for our bodies. Because of the compounds being released into our environment, studies have indicated that the ozone layer in the stratosphere, that absorbs ultraviolet rays from the sun, is being depleted, thereby removing much of the protection from the sun that we previously enjoyed. Twenty to thirty minutes a day of direct sunlight is all that is necessary to promote a healthy body.

If you must be in direct sunlight for an extended period of time, wear shading hats, loose fitting, long sleeved shirts and pants. Use minimal sunblock, as the majority of these products are made from damaging chemicals, which readily absorb into the skin. I have located a reputable company that uses safer ingredients in their sunblock and other personal care products (see Life Changing Products). While people need as much clean, fresh air as possible, minimal sun exposure is best, due to the diets we maintain, as well as the depletion of the ozone layer.

While sunglasses help our eyes adjust to sunlight, the positive effects of sunlight on the body is believed to be transmitted through our eyes to the pineal gland. Some experts believe that wearing glasses that block full-spectrum transmission may reduce some of the health benefits of sun exposure. A balance must be found between risks and benefits of wearing sunglasses. Please consult your own physician for assistance in making an informed and conscious choice concerning sun exposure.

> Note: Consult a doctor if you notice any skin growths or changes. Changes in the coloring of moles and liver spots may indicate problems. In many cases, a biopsy of the affected area can determine if further treatment is needed. More serious measures may be necessary if skin cancers are not caught in time. Early diagnosis is crucial.

~

MOTIVATIONAL TIP

Make it a practice to get outside every day. Lunch is a good time to be outside as many people only receive thirty minutes for lunch. Keep a journal entering information describing how you feel after a few minutes of sunshine. Take a brisk walk, practicing your breathing at the same time. You will see a dramatic difference in your attitude and health.

~

"The great use of life is to spend it for something that will outlast us."
- Charles Mayes

21

REST / SLEEP

The Slumbering Giant

Human sleep is perhaps one of the least understood physiological processes. Its value to human health and proper functioning is without question, absolutely essential to both the body and mind. Sleep is a biological state that is caused by the discharge of specific neurons in certain parts of the brain. It involves an alternate cycle of NREM (Non-Rapid Eye Movement), and REM (Rapid Eye Movement). The cycle consists of 80 minutes of NREM followed by 10 minutes of REM. This 90-minute cycle is repeated from 3 to 6 times during the night.

Getting enough sleep is a major factor in a person's state of health. Sleep is an essential part of the daily routine. Proper sleep allows the body a time to physically and psychologically repair, replenish, and restore itself.

Impaired sleep, altered sleep patterns, and sleep deprivation impair mental and physical function. Many health conditions, particularly depression, chronic fatigue syndrome and fibromyalgia are either entirely or partially related to sleep deprivation or disturbed sleep. Lack of sleep increases susceptibility to illness. I am sure you can recall when a good night's sleep nipped an illness in the bud and restored normal health.

Approximately 39 percent of Americans experience insomnia on a regular basis, with 20 percent claiming that insomnia is a major problem in their lives. Many people use prescription or over-the-counter drugs to treat insomnia. Insomnia is usually nothing more than a symptom of underlying problems such as depression, anxiety, poor digestion, tension, or allergies. It can be brought on by a simple change in daily routine, traveling, starting a new job, going to the doctor or hospital, etc. Various foods, drinks and medications can also cause sleeplessness. It may also be related to more serious health problems. The most effective treatment is to identify the cause and then address it, rather than turning to drug therapy. If drug therapy is used at all, it should be temporary and monitored closely by your physician. Be sure to read the warning labels, as there are many side effects to these medications, especially when mixed with other prescription drugs, alcohol, or certain herbs.

Exactly how much sleep a person requires varies with each individual. Sleep needs tend to decrease with age. A 12-month-old child requires approximately 14 hours of sleep per day, a 6-year-old child about 12 hours, and adults about 7 to 8 hours. Women tend to require more sleep than men do. As we age, our sleep needs may decline but so does our ability to sustain sleep. Decreased levels of brain chemicals such as serotonin and melatonin usually cause this.

¤¤¤

Although insomnia seems to be an ongoing battle for many people there are certain steps we can take to help improve the length and quality of our sleep patterns.

✓ See a doctor and get a thorough examination, both physically and mentally. The need to eliminate serious health conditions is vital. Ask your doctor to check for vitamin and mineral defencies as well. Many people experiencing sleep problems are deficient in calcium and magnesium. Once you have resolved that there are no existing physical health conditions, you need to meet with someone you trust to discuss other mental or emotional problems you may be experiencing.

✓ Sleep on a quality constructed and firm bed. This is essential for entire body support, as well as keeping the spine in alignment.

✓ Go to bed at the same time each day. Our forefathers didn't have alarm clocks to wake them up in the morning. Early on, they didn't even have any type of lighting system and they certainly didn't deal with daylight savings time or working the third shift. They went to bed when the sun went down and got up when the sun came up. We need to do everything possible to replicate the sleep cycles of our forefathers. Strive to go to bed earlier and earlier each evening until you wake up on your own without the aid of an alarm clock. Studies indicate every hour of sleep before midnight equals two, after. So if you feel your day can't end until 11p.m. because of all you have to accomplish, you should go to bed at 9p.m. and get up earlier in the morning to finish your work.

✓ Detoxify your body. A toxic body cannot rest properly. This is the first step in achieving total health.

✓ Exercise every day! We need to be physically tired to rest well. However do not exercise within two hours prior to going to bed. Your body needs time to wind down and relax. This will make a huge difference in the quality and quantity of sleep required (see Chapter 22).

✓ Do not eat within two hours prior to going to bed. Digesting food is the hardest work your body can do. When you eat and go to sleep, the digestion process continues to work. The body heals best when at rest and should not be burdened with digestive tasks at that time. That is why so many people eat, go to bed and fall asleep immediately, only to wake up two hours later and never return to sleep for the night. Once your body completes the digestion process it is ready to continue on with normal daily activities. We have in essence confused our bodily cycles.

✓ Keep the temperature in your bedroom cool, from 60 to 65 degrees, with lots of fresh air. Fresh non-filtered air could pose problems for those with seasonal allergies to pollens and molds. Even if you are allergic, your bedroom should be ventilated with fresh air for at least one hour per day. After the stale, toxic air has been removed and fresh air brought in, run a high efficiency air cleaner to remove any airborne particles. Every bedroom should have a high quality air cleaner operating while sleeping. After all, you spend one-third of your life in the bedroom and it is important that you are breathing pure air.

✓ Keep the bedroom dark and quiet when sleeping. If you need soft music to help you fall to sleep, make sure that the volume is low and that the unit can turn itself off when the music has finished. If you have to get up or roll over to turn it off, you can easily activate your mind and body and have problems falling back to sleep.

✓ Use your bed for sleep and sex. Do not eat, read, knit, watch television or do any other activity in your bed.

✓ Do not allow animals in your bedroom. They carry parasites, which can cause terrible health problems in humans (see Chapter 11). Animals also have dander, which causes allergic reactions in many people.

✓ Indoor plants improve the quality of air. Keep green plants such as a spider plant in your bedroom. Do not keep the plant too damp as mold spores can accumulate and become airborne.

✓ Your bedroom should be free of all toxic materials or articles that collect dust or moisture. The bedding should be 100 percent cotton. No polyester or other chemically derived materials should be used. Your mattress should be wrapped in high quality barrier cloth, as should your pillows. This will prevent dust mites from collecting in your bedding. All bedding should be laundered weekly. All carpets should be removed and hardwood floors, tile or laminate flooring installed. Carpets are breeding places for dust, dust mites and molds. Any dust collecting objects such as knick-knacks, wall hangings, etc., should be removed. Your bedroom should be the least cluttered room in your home. If you have plastic blinds, replace them with metal blinds. When the heat from the sun or the heater comes in contact with the plastic they emit formaldehyde fumes into the air. Do not sleep in a room where dry cleaned clothing is stored. Do not use electric blankets or any electrical device near your bed, such as a digital clock, radio, etc. They should be at least ten feet from the bed, preferably not in the room at all.

✓ Ensure that your bedroom is not located over a crawl space. If it is, be sure to have the dirt floor covered in plastic and also seal the underside of the floor in plastic to keep mold from seeping through the floors and walls. If you go to bed feeling good and wake up feeling sick, this is a good indication that something in the environment is making you ill. Mold is becoming a huge problem in the United States, causing illnesses, forcing people to vacate their residences. This is one reason that a high quality air cleaner should be running continuously in your bedroom.

✓ Sleep on your back. This is the best position for relaxing, and allows all your internal organs to rest properly. If you must sleep on your side, do it on your right side, not your left. Sleeping on the left side causes your lungs, stomach and liver to press against your heart. Never sleep on your stomach. It causes pressure on all your internal organs, especially your lungs, which causes shallow breathing. It can also cause a stiff neck and upper back problems.

✓ Experiment with herbal teas. There are several different herbs that can cause you to relax, allowing you to fall to sleep. Herbs do not in any way react like sleeping pills. You will remain in a normal state of mind and not in some drugged daze. They will not cause memory lapses, nor do they normally cause any kind of hangover feeling in the morning. Some herbs that will cause you to relax are valerian, chamomile, lemon balm, fennel, oat straw, catnip, kava kava, skullcap, passionflower, as well as others. Research and experiment to see what combinations work well for you. Drink the teas about 30 to 45 minutes prior to your bedtime. Treat these herbs as you would medicine and follow the directions on the bottle or those obtained from a qualified herbalist. Too much <u>kava kava</u> can cause stupor and too much <u>valerian</u> will actually cause insomnia. Allow your physician to test you for allergies to these herbs as well.

✓ Take a warm (not hot), relaxing bath. Add one cup of baking soda and one cup of epsom salts and lay back and relax for at least thirty minutes. This mixture will also draw toxins out of your body. Make sure you rinse the soda and epsom salts off with clean, warm water after you bathe.

✓ A massage before bedtime can make many people fall off to sleep in no time at all. Allow a loved one to give slow, gentle yet firm massaging strokes over your body. Make sure you are in bed and ready to go to sleep so that once the message begins you do not have to get up for any reason.

✓ Meditate upon those things that give you peace and a warm, secure feeling. Wind down your evening with a few minutes of inspirational reading, prayer or other forms of relaxation.

✓ Remember your body heals when it sleeps and draws upon your energy when awake. You can eat all the proper foods, exercise daily, meditate, and drink teas but your body can't realize the benefit from these steps unless it is allowed to sleep undisturbed.

~

MOTIVATIONAL TIPS

I remember going days without sleep while I was still trying to hold down a job and run a household. My vision was blurred and my balance unstable. I walked around totally drained every day. After I cleaned out my body, gave it proper nutrition as well as following the steps outlined in this book, I slowly began to improve my sleep patterns. I now have from 7 to 8 hours of uninterrupted sleep each night. I awake refreshed and ready to take on the world. You can too!

Begin pampering yourself each and every evening using the above methods and begin experiencing a good night's rest.

~

"Rest is not idleness, and to lie sometimes on the grass on a summer day listening to the murmur of water or watching the clouds float across the sky, is hardly a waster of time."
- Sir J. Lubbock

Your Thoughts

22

EXERCISE

Essential Movements

Exercise is a key factor in maintaining proper health. Proper cardio-vascular health, musculo-skeletal health, mental health, and the health of the immune system are all greatly improved by a routine exercise regimen. When an insufficient supply of oxygen is received the blood moves sluggishly. The waste, which should be thrown off in the exhalations from the lungs, is retained and the blood becomes impure. Whatever the physical ailment, most all humans can perform some form of exercise. Whether you are bedridden or running a marathon, exercise is vital to your overall performance.

You may eat the most nutritious foods, swear off cigarettes and alcohol and think only positive thoughts, but if you don't exercise, you will never reach the state of optimum health you seek.

Exercise does not promise you eternal youth, but if your body is not moving, you are not alive. We become complacent and bored, and a bored person is boring. One way out of this predicament is to increase your body awareness and viability—exercise! Exercise releases repressed energy and aggressions, enabling us to experience a more restful and sound sleep. It also assists the body in utilizing the nutrients from the foods we eat, thereby improving the digestion process.

Fitness is a lifelong commitment, but physical benefits of getting fit and staying that way are numerous. Exercise firms muscles, strengthens the heart and lungs, improves blood circulation, builds strength and endurance, burns off excess calories, strengthens bones, limbers up the joints, improves digestion, and relieves constipation. Exercise is also beneficial for the mind. It relieves brain weariness, helping us to think more clearly and to feel more cheerful.

Remember that warming up with stretching exercises is very important and equally important is a cool-down. The cool-down allows the heart rate to decrease gradually, as it is very dangerous to suddenly stop after vigorous exercise. It also significantly reduces the build up of lactic acid, which causes cramps, sore muscles and pain.

Also remember, before beginning any exercise program, consult a physician. Having a pre-exercise check-up is a great opportunity to understand where you should begin, assisting you in charting your progress. Exercise, like all other daily activities, must be done with care, thoughtfulness and common sense.

One of the most beneficial forms of exercising is the mini-trampoline. The constant bouncing motion activates the lymphatic system unlike any other physical movement. This motion serves as an internal chelator that pulls toxins out of the tissues and muscles into the blood stream, allowing them to be candidates for elimination. The elimination of these toxins is performed via breathing, perspiration, urination, and bowel elimination.

People who are employed in physically demanding jobs, such as roofers, carpenters, construction workers, etc., have a healthy lymphatic flow.

The mini-trampoline is inexpensive and can be found at most sporting goods stores. People limited by their range of motion can utilize this device as well. Have someone assist the candidate onto the trampoline, in a seated position. The candidate must then attempt to bounce up and down. Many of the same benefits derived from standing and bouncing can be attained from sitting and bouncing. Always be sure to have attendants present during the mounting, utilization, and dismounting of the device.

For people with limited bodily movement, stretching and isometrics are very good exercises. Someone who is bedridden can exercise by writing the alphabet in the air, utilizing their toes. Upon getting tired, rest until later in the day or the next day. Try getting one letter farther everyday. Before long, the entire alphabet will be performed with toe writing. Don't forget both legs need exercising.

Walking briskly is an excellent form of exercise. The pace should be such that having a discussion with a person walking with you would be very difficult. An easily understood conversation is evidence that the pace is not quick enough for a good cardiovascular workout. Use a rhythmic gait that takes the foot from heel to toe, allowing the arms to swing naturally. Do not carry anything on your back or in your arms that will unbalance your body weight. Walking up hill is an excellent addition to the exercise regimen. This extra activity will assist in moving toxins out of the muscles, into the bloodstream. Walking in the country is much preferred over walking in the city, as the air is much more pure and the general environment being more peaceful and healing. Walk on grass or packed dirt, avoiding concrete whenever possible. DO NOT run or jog on a regular schedule. This act can be damaging to the leg joints and internal organs. The continuous pounding shocks the human body, causing your body to experience foot, knee, hip, and internal organ problems.

Swimming, bicycling, gardening, jumping rope, cross-country skiing and mowing the lawn are all excellent forms of exercise. The key to any exercise is to start out slow and easy, making gradual increases. Whenever possible, utilize stairs instead of elevators. Walk to the corner store instead of driving. When shopping, park away from the entrance doors, causing a longer walk to the building.

DO NOT EXERCISE within two hours prior to bedtime. The exercise will stimulate your body causing problems when trying to relax for a restful night of sleep. Morning is the optimum time for exercising as it increases the metabolism and heart rate, allowing the body to burn more calories during the day.

Weight bearing exercises are very beneficial to a continually healthy body. A stronger body more easily burns calories as muscle fibers utilize more caloric energy than fat. A stronger body also helps keep the bones stronger and thicker for a longer period of time. This action will help to fight the onset of osteoporosis.

REMEMBER that the idea is not quantity of weight, but quality of form. Instead of increasing weight, try increasing the repetitions first, reducing the risk of injury due to excessive weight being used. Just about anything easily handled can be used for weight training. Items such as small bags of water, sand, or canned goods work well. A huge expense need not be tied to the exercise.

Increases in any exercise should be gradual, building the cardio-vascular system and the musculo-skeletal system. This will help pull toxins into the bloodstream and speed up transit of the organs of elimination. The objective is long-term health, not short-term results. Keep in mind, it took most of us years to get the bodies we have. Do not expect to transform them overnight.

The utilization of music can be a great addition to an exercise routine. The music will help to keep you in rhythm as well as promote a sense of well being. Select music that will keep you positive, and in a hopeful frame of mind.

Exercise is an integral part of your recovery process.

KEEP MOVING ....KEEP DETOXIFYING

~

MOTIVATIONAL TIPS

When ill, I was able to bounce only twelve times on the trampoline before becoming totally exhausted, needing to return to bed. Within two months, I had worked up to one thousand bounces per day. If I can do it, you can too! I was also unable to walk any distance without assistance. Within a few months, I was able to walk three miles in record time!

I also completed a home study course on the lymphatic system offered by C. Samuel West D.N., N.D. This course was an eye opening experience for me. His simple formulas of "oxygen pumps electricity and power" are five very powerful words. Dr. West is listed in the Resource Guide and his book, *The Golden Seven Plus One*, is listed in the Bibliography in the back of this book. I encourage you to call to take the course.

~

"It is our attitude at the beginning of a difficult undertaking which more than anything else, will determine its outcome."
- William James

23

HERBS & YOUR IMMUNE SYSTEM

Backyard Medicine Chest

The study of herbs affecting the immune system is one of the hottest topics in pharmacological research. Can herbs really strengthen our resistance and help us lead healthier lives? The wisdom of centuries of observation and the scrutiny of the scientific laboratory indicate herbs are powerful allies in our fight for good health. Herbalism, the knowledge and study of herbs, may not be a term in your active vocabulary, but is a reality in your life. The mustard on your table, many of the spices in your kitchen, and most of the vegetables in your salad are herbs. An herb is defined as a non-woody plant that dies down to the ground after flowering. The term "herb" is often applied more generally to any plant, or plant part that has been used for such purposes as medical treatment, nutrition, food seasoning, coloring or dyeing of other substances.

For most of man's existence, various but limited resources were available for the treatment of injuries and disease. Plants were the basic source of therapeutic products for professional and folk medicine from the earliest days, until the twentieth century. Plant remedies represent the most continuous and universal form of treatment.

The twentieth century has not been kind to old knowledge and traditions, including those of herbalism. Modern ideas and techniques have largely replaced herbal remedies. Synthetic drugs, processed foods, plant dyes, and colorings by chemical substitutes have replaced natural remedies. Even common sense and self-reliance have been replaced by deference to authority and lack of self-confidence. However, a renewed interest in herbalism exists. The utilization of herbs in Europe and proven facts from scientific studies has forced the United States to recognize the effectiveness of alternative medical treatment.

Acknowledgment of plants concerning their usefulness in medicine is becoming more prevalent. New plants are continuously being investigated for therapeutic properties. Did you know that—quinine is derived from cinchona bark; morphine from the opium poppy; digitalis from foxglove; the tranquilizer reserpine from rauwolfia, and ephedrine from ma-huang?

¤¤¤

Listed below is a small portion of the many plants that can aid in building the immune system as well as treat illnesses that have already established themselves within the body.

- **Alfalfa**: Plants have been known to reach as much as thirty feet deep into the soil. The leaves of the plant are rich in minerals and nutrients, including calcium, magnesium, potassium and carotene. They are also a source of protein, Vitamin E and Vitamin K. Alfalfa has been used in Chinese medicine since the sixth

century to treat kidney stones, an(
retention and swelling. It also nouri:
skeletal, glandular, and urinary
contains chlorophyll, which is 1
cleansing qualities. <u>Chlorophyll</u> is a
want to forget. You can obtain :
colored foods. It is a powerhouse
cleansing.

- **Aloe Vera**: Historically known
functions of the gastrointestinal
properties of soothing, cleansing, an(
to maintain healthy tissues. This pla:
of facilitating digestion, aiding blo
circulation, as well as kidney, live
functions. It contains at least three
fatty acids that are helpful for tl
intestine and colon. It naturally :
juices to prevent excessive amounts
discovered compound in aloe, acem
being studied for its ability to strer
system. Studies have shown acem
lymphocyte cells that aid natural resi

- **Angelica Root**: Nutritionally sup|
and respiratory systems. Calmin;
system.

- **Anise**: Seeds act to remove exc
gastrointestinal tract.

- **Barberry**:* Nourishes the liver a
helps the bile to flow freely. It h
from the bowel.

ayberry:* Excellent blood purifier and detoxifier. ffective for helping to stop a cold from forming if ken when the first symptoms appear.

ack Cohosh:* The root is used to ease complaints sociated with the skeletal system. Traditionally used r many gynecological topics, including menstrual amps, and menstruation. Black Cohosh is also used to lm the nervous system by nourishing blood vessels, d balancing the hormones in menopausal women. udies show it contains substances that bind to trogen receptors.

ack Walnut:* The hulls contain a substance which lps the body eliminate parasites. It is also used for ison oak, ringworm and skin ailments. It has tifungal properties and is also said to promote bowel ;ularity. (Can be used externally while pregnant.)

rdock: A natural blood purifier and detoxifier. It is 'ored for helping the body maintain healthy skin. It urishes the urinary and respiratory systems, and also tritionally supports joints and other skeletal tissues.

scara Sagrada:* Used to help the body relieve istipation. Also reputed for nutritionally supporting stomach, liver, pancreas, and gallbladder. It is ansing, as well as nourishing, to the colon, however, uld be used infrequently.

tnip: Nourishes the stomach and nerves. An old e favorite drink to relax and help promote a good hts sleep.

- **Cat's Claw:*** Known to help nutritionally support the body's immune, circulatory, urinary tract and gastrointestinal systems through its antioxidant and building properties. This prevents the bacteria from spreading and eventually results in the halt of infection.

- **Dandelion**: Powerfully nourishes the liver and contains many vital nutrients. Has been used traditionally to purify the blood and to benefit the circulatory and glandular systems.

- **Dong Quai:*** Stimulates the central nervous system and nourishes the brain. It also balances and strengthens female organs and regulates their functions. Acts as a blood tonic and laxative.

- **Echinacea**: Modern scientific studies now validate Echinacea's traditional usage as a topical agent to help the body repair skin wounds, and internally enhance the immune system. The active constituents in the plant are thought to bolster the body's defense system and are known as polysaccharides. Polysaccharides stimulate the activity of macrophages, white blood cells that destroy bacteria, viruses, other invaders, and even wayward cells. It also activates the body's production of interferon, a specific protein that protects cells against the invasion of viruses.

- **Fennel**: Helps to detoxify and remove waste material from the body.

- **Fenugreek**: This herb has many traditional uses, including nourishing the skin, respiratory system, and the pancreas. It helps the body to expel mucus and toxins. It also dissolves fat and is high in nutrients.

- **Flax Seed Oil**: Provides omega 3 (linolenic acid), omega 6, and omega 9 fatty acids. Omegas 3 and 6 benefit the cardio-vascular system, as well as the immune and nervous systems. It also contains some beta carotene and Vitamin E.

- **Garlic**: Provides nourishment for the circulatory, immune and urinary systems. It aids in supporting with normal circulation, nourishing stomach tissues, maintaining normal blood pressure and aids the body's natural ability to resist disease. Garlic is a natural antibiotic and fungicide. <u>An herb no home should be without</u>!

- **Ginger**: Nourishing to the gastrointestinal system. It also helps the body to eliminate wastes through the skin. It enhances circulation and acts as a catalyst for other herbs, increasing their effectiveness. It relieves the body of congestion. It is also used for nausea.

- **Ginkgo Biloba:*** Effective in nutritionally supporting the body's system, especially through its antioxidant properties. Ginkgo is a very potent free radical scavenger. Eliminating free radicals is important in preserving youthfulness. The Orient has long valued this herb for its effect on the challenges of aging.

- **Ginseng**: Beneficial for the immune system and energy. It nourishes the circulatory system and enhances mental alertness and stamina. Long-term use can lead to hormone balance problems and may promote nervousness and premature ejaculation. Siberian Ginseng is milder than American Ginseng.

- **Golden Seal:*** Used both internally and externally to help the body fight infections with its nutritional properties. It helps the body soothe inflammations of the mucous membranes and balance their function. This herb especially nourishes the liver, glandular and respiratory systems. It also helps to cleanse the system of foreign organisms. <u>Note</u>: Can initiate miscarriage.

- **Hops**: Helps the body with pain and insomnia. Hops are rich in nutrients that nourish the nervous system. Considered a tonic and relaxant.

- **Horehound Leaf (White)**: Soothing to the respiratory system and is a natural expectorant.

- **Horehound (Black)**: Is used for nausea and vomiting and should not be confused with White Horehound.

- **Horsetail:*** This herb is rich in nutrients that support the nails, skin, hair, bones and the body's connective tissue. It also benefits the glands and urinary tract.

- **Hydrangea:*** Traditionally used to strengthen the urinary tract and help regulate its function. This plant contains alkaloids that help soothe the body, especially in the bladder and kidney areas. It works like a natural inflammation reliever and cleanses the joint areas.

- **Hyssop**: Used for hundreds of years as an herbal remedy for afflictions of the respiratory system. It soothes throats and nourishes the lungs.

- **Kava Kava:*** Soothes the nerves and pain relief. Too much can cause stupor. <u>Note</u>: Use with caution.

- **Kelp**: Contains nearly thirty minerals that nourish the thyroid and pituitary glands. It helps balance the body's metabolism and rate at which it burns calories. It is also known as seaweed, growing in the rich ocean beds. It nourishes the sensory nerves, brain membranes, spinal cord and brain tissue. Kelp contains alginic acid, which can help protect the body against the effects of radiation.

- **Licorice:*** Nutritionally supports the respiratory system, gastrointestinal system, heart and spleen. This herb can soothe irritated mucus membranes and help the body rid itself of unwanted mucus with its expectorant properties. Licorice Root has properties similar to cortisone and estrogen. It stimulates the adrenal glands and helps the body cope with stress. <u>Note</u>: Not to be used by those with water retention, high blood pressure or excessive hair growth.

- **Lobelia:*** Possesses soothing properties that nourish the nervous system. Enhances the function of the respiratory system and has antispasmodic effects. <u>Note</u>: 1) Must be used in very small amounts, as it is toxic in low dosages and will cause vomiting. 2) Use only under practitioner's care.

- **Mandrake:*** Supports the liver, gallbladder and digestion in general. It has a powerful influence on the glands. <u>Note</u>: Very toxic. Use only under practitioners care.

- **Marshmallow**: Possesses soothing properties and nutritionally supports the respiratory, urinary and gastrointestinal systems.

- **Milk Thistle**: The extract is a potent antioxidant, which prevents harm from free radicals and lends nutritional support to the liver. The seed extract contains silymarin; a unique type of flavonoid-like compound considered the active ingredient in Milk Thistle.

- **Mullein**: Traditionally referred to as a "natural wonder herb" which soothes the lungs and irritations associated within the respiratory tract. It also nourishes the lymphatic and glandular systems. Mullein can assist in moving mucus from the systems.

- **Myrrh**:* The resin soothes muscles and wounds. Nourishes mucus membranes with its cleansing effects. May also be used as a gargle and mouthwash. Should be administered in small doses only.

- **Nettles**: A safe daily tonic full of chlorophyll, vitamins and minerals. It tones and supports all organ systems, aids in elimination and works particularly well with allergies of all kinds.

- **Noni**:* Very popular plant today that helps support the body's respiratory, immune, digestive and structural systems.

- **Parsley**:* Blood builder, cleanser and has blood pressure regulating properties.

- **Pau d'Arco:*** A South American herb with anti-fungal properties that helps strengthen and nourish the body's defense system. A healthy immune system is a key in fighting diseases and infections.

- **Passionflower**: Helps to reduce anxiety, hysteria and nervousness by nourishing the nervous system. Used for pain, insomnia, nervous exhaustion, asthma and attention deficit disorder. In vitro experiments show that passicol, an alkaloid found in passionflower, kills a range of molds, yeasts, and bacteria.

- **Peppermint**: Calms the stomach, intestinal tract, and nervous system. Peppermint is a wonderful tea to drink alone or mixed with less palatable herbs. Promotes sweating during colds and flu.

- **Red Clover**: A great general immune tonic. Brings on a normal menstrual cycle, promotes fertility, balances hormones associated with menopausal symptoms. Has important vitamins and minerals.

- **Red Raspberry Leaf**: Strengthens the wall of the uterus and regulates menstrual flow. It nourishes the reproductive organs, especially the uterine muscles, and helps strengthen and prepare the body for childbirth. It is soothing and also has astringent properties to the stomach and intestinal tract. This herb also strengthens the heart muscle. A nutrient rich herb that helps balance the body so that diarrhea or constipation can be alleviated. Especially good for children and adults recovering from a prolonged illness.

- **Rhubarb**:* Dissolves mucus adhering to the walls of the colon.

- **Safflower**: The flowers of the safflower plant are used to nourish the liver, gallbladder and respiratory system. Safflower helps balance cholesterol in the body, and assists in eliminating excessive uric acid. It helps break up phlegm and soothes the digestive system.

- **Sage**:* Eliminates excessive mucus in the body. <u>Note</u>: Lactating women should not use, as it tends to dry up the milk.

- **Saw Palmetto**: The berry is said to nourish glandular tissue, and has been used to nutritionally support the prostate gland.

- **Skullcap**: Powerful, yet gentle herb promoting a good night's sleep. It calms the nervous system, relaxes the muscles, and helps balance blood pressure.

- **Senna**:* Expels wastes from the intestines and kills worms.

- **Slippery Elm**: Assists the body in eliminating mucus from the lungs and strengthens the gastrointestinal and respiratory systems. It soothes irritated tissues and helps nourish and strengthen the body.

- **Suma**:* Suma is an adaptogen herb, which means it helps the body adapt to stress, and acts as a tonic to the entire system. It enhances the immune system, preventing free-radical damage to the body. Suma contains significant amounts of germanium, a trace mineral that stimulates the immune system and helps to promote oxygen flow to the cells. It contains "allantoin," a substance that assists in healing wounds. It also has a good supply of vitamins, minerals, essential amino acids, and the natural plant hormones sitosterol and stigmasterol. These phytochemicals nourish the circulatory and glandular systems.

- **Thyme**:* Powerful antiseptic and general tonic. It has been used in cases of bronchial and intestinal disturbances.

- **Uva Ursi**:* Strengthens the urinary system and helps the body eliminate excess water.

- **Valerian**:* Nourishes the nervous system and has soothing properties being used as a natural sleep aid. Calms muscles, nerves, and blood vessels. Note: Overdose can actually cause insomnia.

- **Watermelon Seeds**: Used as a diuretic in eliminating excess water from the body.

- **Wild Yam**:* It is known to relax the muscles and promote glandular balance in women. Contains natural plant components called phytochemicals, which help the body balance hormone levels. Nourishes nerves and digestive system.

- **Wormwood**:* Eliminates worms and parasites.

- **Yellow Dock**: A bitter herb noted for its high iron content. Nourishes the skin, stimulates bile production, tones the liver and gallbladder, and purifies the blood. Also has a mild laxative effect.

*Avoid during pregnancy.

This is just a sampling of the many herbs available to us. Many different herbs help heal the same system within the body. Therefore, if one specific herb is not available, other herbs may have the same healing qualities.

~

MOTIVATIONAL TIPS

Many people believe if "a little is good, then more must be better." This is not true with herbs. Herbs are powerful and should be treated with respect. Research and educate yourself before using herbs. Find a respected Herbalist to direct and instruct you about the utilization of herbs (see Resource Guide). There is a multitude of wonderful herb books on the market. Every home needs a comprehensive and illustrated herbal guide.

Contact someone who has knowledge with herbs and take a stroll through your backyard or woods. You will be amazed at the many medicinal plants you have available to you. Learn how to grow, dry, and store herbs. Experiment with the many unusual tastes of herbs. Make teas, spring tonics, tinctures, decoctions, syrups and juices of these wonderful plants.

188 DYING IN THE LAND OF PLENTY

While seriously ill, my liver and kidneys were barely functioning. I began using a powerful product that included milk thistle, dandelion root and other herbs (see Life Changing Products). It assisted in bringing health to my liver and kidneys which prescription drugs were unable to do. The problems I have overcome utilizing herbs are a statement to the power they possess.

Isn't it nice to know you have a medicine chest in your backyard?

~

"The purpose of life is to be useful, to be honorable, to be compassionate, to have it make some difference that you have lived and lived well."

- Ralph Waldo Emerson

24

CHIROPRACTIC

Align Me

Chiropractic science teaches that the health of the spine is essential to the health of the body. The brain and spinal nerves control and coordinate the function of all the tissues, organs and systems in the body. Our brain and spinal cord are fairly well protected within our skull and spinal column. However, the nerves that leave the spinal column to connect with our muscles and organs, called spinal nerves, are not as well protected. When the nerves become compressed between the joints of our spine, we can experience pain. Pain is our body's way of telling us something is wrong and needs attention.

Although the design of the spine is quite splendid, incorporating flexibility, strength and resilience in its critical role of protecting the spinal cord, our daily activities at times take their toll on this jointed vertebra. The spine is susceptible to the stress and strain of everyday life and may, at times, require professional attention. Extending from the skull to the pelvis and formed of 24 vertebrae and 122 joints, the human spine is an engineering marvel. Along with 300 muscles and 375 ligaments, the spine supports the head, trunk, upper limbs and itself, while transferring the weight of the body to the lower limbs. The spine also houses and protects the spinal cord and the thirty-one pairs of spinal nerves which branch from the spinal cord and travel through openings between the vertebrae, called intervertebral foramen, to the rest of the body.

Many people experience chiropractic as a natural drug-free way to improve health. This practice is used to treat back or neck pain, digestion problems, colic, bed-wetting, headache, sciatica, asthma as well as a host of other symptoms. People also visit their chiropractor for increased energy, improved sports performance and a general, all-around immune boosting, therapy session.

When your spine is out of alignment, the brain's ability to communicate with the body is restricted. The body's ability to protect itself is impaired. Chiropractors remove a serious interference in your life and health called vertebral subluxations, which prevent you from functioning at your best. You will be more balanced, with less stress on your nervous system and body structures, after effective treatment has begun.

Insurance companies now recognize chiropractic medicine as being a vital part of our overall health. This is a big step in alternative medicine and goes hand-in-hand with traditional medicine.

~

MOTIVATIONAL TIPS

Chiropractic procedures can play a vital part in your overall health. Choose a Chiropractor that is willing to work closely with your healthcare provider as well as yourself, when implementing a complete protocol for you to follow, resulting in your renewed health.

Not all practitioners use the same methods. Research and ask for referrals. Once you begin treatment be sure to follow instructions closely and give yourself ample time to feel the results (see Resource Guide).

~

"The greater part of our happiness or misery depends on our dispositions and not our circumstances."

- Martha Washington

Your Thoughts

25

HOMEOPATHY

Treating "Like With Like"

The term "homeopathy" is derived from the Greek words *homeos* meaning similar, and *pathos,* meaning disease. A state of homeostasis, physiologic balance, is a primary goal of homeopathy, a system of natural medicine developed in the late 1700s by the German physician, Samuel Hahnemann. Hahnemann was seeking a kinder, gentler alternative to the often harsh treatments of his day. He argued that any substance that produces a symptom in a healthy person could cure that symptom in a sick person. In large part, he attained his goal. In fact, by the late 1800s there were 110 homeopathic hospitals and 145 homeopathic dispensaries in the United States, successfully treating typhoid fever, yellow fever, cholera, and other diseases of the time that carried a significant mortality rate. Hahnemann challenged the medical establishment of his time, starting a running battle that continues today. When modern medicine and the pharmaceutical industry emerged in this century during the early 1900s, their politicking all but destroyed homeopathic practice. Nevertheless, homeopathy's popularity abroad remained strong. Its growing reputation in England, where it has been incorporated into the British national health system, as well as in Europe, Greece, India, Mexico, and Argentina, has helped fuel its current renaissance in the United States.

A homeopathic remedy is a microdilution or microdose of the very same plant, mineral, or chemical substance that, in its original concentration, will bring on that illness. For instance, ipecac syrup induces nausea and vomiting, while homeopathic ipecac diminishes nausea and vomiting. Thus homeopathy embodies the principle of "like curing like."

Equally fascinating is the fact that the weaker the dilution, thus the smaller the microdose, the stronger and deeper-acting the remedy. In fact, the most diluted remedies have no detectable original active ingredient left. Modern homeopathic mixtures can be diluted a millionfold or more! The "essence" or energy of the substance creates its effect. Such concepts defy conventional medical understanding, which is why they engender much skepticism toward homeopathic practice.

¤¤¤

Homeopathic remedies have several distinct advantages over conventional drug therapy:

- They are non-toxic in effect and rarely cause any harm.

- They affect healing at deeper levels than the superficial suppression of symptoms common to conventional drug therapy, making them extremely useful in the treatment of chronic conditions.

- They are ideal for infants, children and pets who cannot swallow pills, or who dislike the taste of many medications or herbs.

- They can be effective when other alternative approaches have failed, and for illnesses that are thought to be "untreatable."

¤¤¤

A correctly prescribed homeopathy remedy will trigger a defense response, stimulate heightened vitality, and bring an individual back to health. By restoring balance and strength at physical, mental, and emotional levels, homeopathy can affect true cures, because the whole individual is being treated.

Homeopathy differs from conventional medicine in that it treats the individual with the disease as a whole rather than the disease alone. Herein lies one of the reasons for homeopathy's success.

~

MOTIVATIONAL TIPS

Remember, what works for one person may not work for another. Become familiar with this type of treatment. Homeopathy lends itself extremely well to self-care, particularly in cases of common illnesses and injuries.

Learn to treat minor problems before they require medical intervention. After you become more knowledgeable about different remedies, your confidence will increase and the process becomes easier. Knowing the remedy is the key. All this will require time, patience and learning.

Visit your local library or bookstore. There is much information available on this subject.

~

"Difficult times have helped me understand better than before, how infinitely rich and beautiful life is in every way, and that so many things that one goes worrying about are of no importance whatsoever."

- Isak Dinesen

26

MORE NATURAL THERAPEUTICS

The Road Less Traveled

Bee Venom Therapy has been used for centuries as a natural anti-inflammatory for chronic pain and degenerative diseases. Much research has taken place in Russia, Austria, Germany, France, England, Switzerland and Czechoslovakia regarding this simple therapy. Many patients have successfully utilized bee venom as therapy for the following conditions:

- Acute and Chronic Rheumatoid Arthritis
- Acute and Chronic Osteoarthritis
- Bursitis
- Fibromyalgia
- Fibrositis
- Gout
- Multiple Sclerosis
- Neuralgia
- Neuritis
- Rheumatism
- Tendonitis

Bee venom contains several biologically active components that simulate the pituitary-adrenal axis to release both adrenaline and cortisol. Cortisol is one of the body's most potent anti-inflammatory substances.

Most health practitioners utilizing bee venom therapy give their patients injections from multiple-dose vials. The venom is scraped from the diaphragm of honeybees. It is then processed, sterilized, and bottled for use. It is sometimes mixed with a local anesthetic and then injected under the skin. Practitioners will always check their patients for bee venom allergy. If no allergy is found, a gradually increasing number of injections are given on a regular schedule. The health practitioner will closely monitor for any reactions to the injections. Some say that collecting the venom in vials, loses some of its potency, but in many situations this is more realistic than finding a beekeeper or handling bees.

> Note: If other types of treatment for the above
> symptoms have proven fruitless, bee venom
> therapy might be a viable option for your
> particular needs. You must consult a
> physician dedicated to understanding and
> administering natural remedies.

Hydrotherapy is the use of water (hot, cold, steam, or ice) in the treatment or prevention of illness dating back to 1500 B.C. Many cultures used hydrotherapy such as the Egyptians, Assyrians, Persians, Hebrews, Hindus, Chinese, and Greeks and it was used extensively by Hippocrates, making it one of the most ancient methods of treatment. Bathhouses were an essential part of ancient Roman culture. Roman physicians Galen and Celsus wrote of treating patients with warm and cold baths in order to prevent disease. Bathhouses made their first appearance in America in the mid-1700s.

Everyone has at some time or other experienced the soothing and relaxing qualities of a hot bath, as well as the invigorating and stimulating effects of a cold shower or swim. Water applications offer an increase in localized white blood cell counts. Hydrotherapy can be beneficial in the treatment of sore throats, colds, bronchitis, pneumonia, abscesses, pelvic inflammatory disease, bladder infections, flu, chronic fatigue syndrome, as well as other conditions.

Because of its effects on circulation and other physiologic parameters, hydrotherapy is also helpful for other bodily ailments. Those include nervous conditions, insomnia, anxiety, acute and chronic pain, poor circulation, headaches, muscle spasms, fever, arthritis, and fatigue. It also aids the prostate, uterus, glandular congestion, and the overall bodily detoxification process.

The heating and cooling effects of water are responsible for its therapeutic benefits. A hot compress can open blood vessels and attract more blood to the area (ex: abscesses). Enhancing the circulation also improves organ function. Hot water is also thought to stimulate the immune system. Moist heat relaxes tense muscles or spasms. Adding Epsom salts and certain herbs can also enhance its effects. A compress of extremely cold water will constrict blood vessels and decrease circulation (useful in treating sprains), reducing inflammation. Cold water works well to diminish pain caused by a congestive condition, such as a vascular headache.

Adding herbs and essential oils to water can enhance its therapeutic value. Steam is frequently used as a carrier for essential oils that are inhaled to treat respiratory problems.

Information may be obtained via the Internet and bookstores. Physicians practicing non-invasive natural healing therapies can identify a plan of treatment for utilizing hydrotherapy.

Massage - It will be rare that you find a person that doesn't enjoy a good massage. Massage therapy has been used for centuries to assist in detoxification, inducing healing. The origins of therapeutic massage are rooted in the common instinctual response to hold and rub a hurt or pain. It is found in all cultures as an integral part of health care. As alternative methods of healing become more prevalent in today's world, massage therapy is regaining its rightful place among health care practitioners. The goal is to teach body awareness and address underlying structural problems.

There are several types of techniques used in massage therapy. The Swedish massage is a relatively gentle technique that can increase circulation of blood to the lymph system, bringing relaxation to tense muscles and nerves. It shortens recovery time from muscular strain by flushing the tissues of lactic acid, uric acid, and other metabolic wastes. Deep tissue massage is the deep and sometimes painful probing of underlying connective tissue and muscle sheaths helping realign posture along true planes of movement. This will assist the body in finding its centerline of gravity, increase efficiency of movements, and relieve many chronic and recurring musculoskeletal conditions.

Craniosacral techniques employed by some chiropractors and osteopaths involve the very gentle and subtle manipulation of the cranial bones and the sacrum. The cranial bones of the skull are movable joints that can be misaligned by trauma from birth, head injury, dental stress, and other factors. Infringing on the brain and the flow of cerebrospinal fluid, such misalignments can cause or contribute to headaches, seizures, behavioral, learning, and visual problems, as well as vertigo. It can also contribute to TMJ (Temporomandibular Joint Dysfunction), spinal, and other musculo-skeletal pain. Craniosacral technique is considered one of the more refined and specialized of the manipulation therapies.

Physical therapy is another form of bodywork long considered an extension of conventional medicine. It is very effective for a variety of musculo-skeletal conditions. This type of massage can be used to prevent muscular atrophy in cases of broken bones, to reduce inflammation in strains and sprains, to increase circulation of varicose ulcers, to stimulate normal bowel movement and much more.

Human beings respond to touch, sometimes quite dramatically. Even without special medical training in these areas, there is much that we as human beings can do for each other. Simply holding someone's hand can bring a feeling of security or trigger a needed emotional release. Rubbing someone's back or neck can ease tense muscles and often put them to sleep. Gently stimulating someone's temple area can relieve a headache. Laying your hands gently on someone's stomach can reduce pain and anxiety. Time has proven that a loving touch can help speed the recovery process.

Ginger Compress - The main purpose of a ginger compress is to strongly increase blood circulation and body fluids at areas where stagnation exists. This stagnation usually manifests itself in the form of pain, inflammation, swelling or stiffness. Used in Japanese traditional healing, a ginger compress can be useful for conditions requiring heat and improved circulation. Examples are sinus inflammation, bronchial and other lung infections, sore throat, and stomach flu. Get specific instructions from your doctor prior to using these compresses as overexposure can burn the skin.

Castor Oil Pack - Castor Oil has been used throughout the ages as a natural therapy. Applied externally in the form of "packs" it is very popular with natural health practitioners. Castor oil packs involve the topical application of castor oil to treat a variety of symptoms and conditions. These include constipation, intestinal toxicity, intestinal and abdominal cramping, liver congestion/sluggishness, ovarian cysts, menstrual cramps, fibroids, hepatitis, tendonitis, bursitis, bruises, plantar warts, varicose veins, bronchitis, pneumonia and more.

There is concrete evidence on the effectiveness of a castor oil pack. Just how and why it works is uncertain. It has been suggested that a certain amount of lymphatic flow or perhaps T-cell stimulation can be the reasons for success. Perhaps an increase in circulation to the treated areas allows for the success of this particular application.

Acupuncture is a component of the health care system of China that can be traced back for at least 2,500 years. As part of the oldest complete medical system, acupuncture probably was used to treat more people than any other method in the history of the world. Stone and iron needles have been found in South America and Egypt, as well as in China, suggesting the use of acupuncture in ancient civilizations. It was not used widely in America until the early 1970s.

Patients who have experienced this treatment describe it as both energizing and deeply relaxing, because it essentially balances and tonifies the nervous system. According to research studies, it regulates the nervous system by increasing the number of blood cells and circulating immune agents and by releasing anti-inflammatory and pain relieving chemicals produced by the body. It is also used in the treatment of nausea and vomiting, pulmonary problems such as asthma and bronchitis and the rehabilitation from neurological damage such as that caused by stroke.

The World Health Organization also recommends the use of acupuncture for conditions such as arthritis, bursitis, tendonitis, back pain, sciatica, neck and shoulder strain, and migraine and tension headaches. It is also been successful in the treatment of impotence, infertility, diabetes and diabetic neuropathy, chronic fatigue, allergies, digestive disorders, bronchitis, urinary incontinence, constipation, depression, insomnia, high blood pressure as well as a host of other ailments.

Acupuncture is a complex intervention that varies for each patient. The number and length of treatments and the specific points used may also vary among individuals.

If you decide to use this approach, research thoroughly and get the credentials of the doctor prior to undergoing the technique administered to you. This information is to raise your awareness of the alternative natural healing techniques available to you. Always consult a physician prior to utilizing any of these techniques.

~

MOTIVATIONAL TIPS

What works for some people will not necessarily work for all. You must experiment with different methods of treatment. If you do experiment please be sure to allow adequate time for the treatment to give effective results.

Remember natural methods do not necessarily work as quickly as drugs in many cases, nor are they as toxic, or symptom masking as drugs.

I personally have used the castor oil compresses, hydrotherapy and massage therapy with great success. I use hydrotherapy, garlic, oregano oil, lemon and honey teas, and fresh juices each time my son contracts a cold or bronchitis. He hasn't been prescribed an antibiotic in over five years. Prior to that he was on a maintenance dose of antibiotics for two years, due to the frequency of infections. Our family is a testimonial to the benefits of building and maintaining the immune system via natural methods.

The massage therapy was also a very instrumental part of my healing. I recommend it highly!

~

"Learn to get in touch with the silence within yourself and know that everything in this life has a purpose."
- Elizabeth Kubler Ross

27

SPIRITUALITY / MEDITATION

Your Lifeline To Good Health

If you have read this book and it has brought you to this section, I assume you are ill, know someone who is, or are interested in the prevention of illness before it affects yourself or your family. Another assumption is that you may be overwhelmed with the entire list of Do's & Don'ts that have been identified throughout this book. You may think, "I am too sick to start doing all this work" or "I am not sick enough and may venture at another time in my life to implement this program." You may even be thinking, "I may at least begin taking some of the measures listed to improve my health or prevent illness from taking a foothold." Whatever you do, do not make the fatal mistake of sitting idle, watching the world go by and do nothing!

As you read this section, closely examine your life. What decisions have you made that have had a negative impact in your life? Are they decisions where the results can never be reversed? Are there steps you can take to correct some of the poor choices you have made? Are there steps you can take to help you adapt or live with the choices you have made? Make a list of the poor choices you feel you have made in your life. Examine each one, taking appropriate time to ponder the choices and the resulting consequences. When you feel comfortable with your thoughts, take appropriate action. For example, apologize to someone you may have hurt physically or emotionally. Talk to someone that may have hurt you, telling them how you felt when it happened and how it affected your life. Maybe, confessing the truth to someone about an instance where you told a lie. How about, returning something that you may have taken that wasn't rightfully yours? It may not have been a material possession that was taken, but someone's innocence or freedom.

The necessary action may be just "letting go" and forgiving someone for any unfairness you felt was done to you. You may never choose to talk to the person or the person may no longer be living. However, you need to put the hurt behind you and start a new life, with new hope. True healing, physical, emotional, and spiritual, can never take place until ill feelings are laid aside. If you need to speak to a counselor or clergy, you should make an appointment immediately. Do not delay, for time is running short. Seize the opportunity to give yourself the blessing of true freedom and hope for the future.

ALL of us live in a world of regrets and "what ifs." This world is not a world of love and peace as originally planned, it is a world that hosts anger, jealously, resentment, greed, hate, war, terrorism, disease, crime, murder, divorce, drugs, physical and mental abuse, and lies. All these negative feelings join forces in an attempt to weaken our bodies to the point of death. Because of the wondrous way we are created, we have choices that can redeem us from this weary lifestyle.

Today is the day to make the correct choice, the only choice that will grant you total peace and true happiness. Vow to spend at least fifteen minutes each morning in quiet solitude thanking God for the situation you are in currently. Ask him to show you what you need to learn by this experience and how you can use it to teach others. After you have communicated with God, listen quietly for his direction. Listen very closely, as he will answer. He may answer in the most unexpected way. Be patient.

Whatever grave circumstances you may be dealing with, realize that God has the power and will give you the power to change or accept those circumstances. Submit yourself to him and ask him for his guidance and direction. Ask him to show you how to rely on him for your decisions. He has promised in his Holy Word to give wisdom to those that ask. Ask, believing and knowing, that you will receive.

In our *Holy Bible*, Hosea 4:6 states, "my people are destroyed for lack of knowledge." I do not claim to have all the knowledge, but God did allow a crisis in my life to occur and I have gained valuable insight. It is now your turn to grow, from gained knowledge, research further, increasing that knowledge, adapt it into your own life and reach out to others. If we are to have true faith in our spouses, our doctors, our children, and ourselves we first must have faith in God. For it is he that is in total control of all circumstances.

If your medical doctor has diagnosed you with a terminal illness, remember that it is God that will determine when you take your last shallow breath on this earth. All things are possible with God. Where there is life, there is hope. Do not give up until God gives you the peace of knowing you are ready to leave this life. If he doesn't give you that peace, then there is work for you to do here and you must fulfill that obligation to truly feel peace and happiness. Others may need your help. Others may need to know what you have experienced, growing and healing from your testimony.

Wherever you find yourself at this point, realize that nothing happens in our lives without our great Creator allowing it to happen. Please understand that I said "allow to happen" not "cause to happen." Therefore, whatever situation you find yourself in at this very moment, it has been allowed. God created us with a free will allowing us to make choices. Many times we put our lives in turmoil, we hurt the people we love the most, we make wrong choices in our marriages, our careers, the discipline of our children, the money we spend, the food we eat, and the habits we keep.

It is our responsibility to use everything available to reverse the wrong choices we have made. Most of us are guilty of starving our bodies of the necessary nutrients needed for good health. We also starve our souls of food necessary to sustain eternal life. In this book you have been given tools to reverse this process. If you team up with God, health care professionals, family and friends, you have power on your side. Remember that all things are possible.

~

MOTIVATIONAL TIPS

Research a topic you have little or no knowledge about. When I was going through my long recovery process, I did extensive research in health, nutrition, environmental toxins, and anything else that I felt may have contributed to my illness.

As I became healthier, I wanted answers as to why God had allowed this terrible experience to happen in my life. I began researching the history of religion, as well as studying scriptures from God's word. As time progressed "things and circumstances" in my life began to make sense. I now look back on that time in my life and realize what a blessing that illness has truly proven to be. I would never again want to relive that agony. However, I can now understand what people mean when they say that they feel so sick, they would like to just give up, lay down and have it all end. I can now empathize with them and give them hope, as I have felt the same feelings.

This illness gave me a whole new appreciation for life as well as the desire to help others understand the cause and prevention of disease, enabling them to live full and healthy lives.

My hope is for you to also learn from the lessons life has taught you, to share and comfort others in their time of distress.

~

"A sad soul can kill you quicker than a germ."

- John Steinbeck

Your Thoughts

28

DO'S & DON'TS

For Health - For Life

DO

- o Listen to your body.

- o Learn the anatomy of your body, understand how it works. Knowing how your body works can help you determine what steps you need to take in maintaining your health.

- o Get a thorough physical from a knowledgeable and qualified physician.

- o Treat all vitamin and mineral deficiencies with high-potency quality supplements and raw, whole foods under the guidance of your physician or other knowledgeable health care provider.

- o Research and experiment with healing herbs (check for allergic reactions).

o   Get out of doors as much as possible (even in bad weather).

o   Get some sunshine every day.

o   Allow fresh air to flow through your house <u>every</u> day.

o   Use high quality air cleaners to purify indoor air.

o   Breathe fresh air, deeply each morning and throughout the day. Learn proper breathing techniques and make them habit.

o   Use correct posture. Don't slouch or cross your legs.

o   Wear cotton clothing. Keep arms and legs as evenly clad as the rest of your body. Don't wear materials labeled "dry clean only."

o   Wear leather or canvas shoes with leather soles (no synthetic materials).

o   Sleep on a firm, comfortable mattress.

o   Concentrate on detoxifying your bedroom first!

o   Keep temperature in bedroom cool (60-65 degrees).

o   Drink lots of pure water, from glass only.

o   Remember to change your water filters often.

o Bathe daily with exfoliating gloves (very warm wash, very cool rinse).

o Keep your nails impeccably clean.

o Take at least two saunas per week, after you are on the road to recovery.

o Exercise daily. Stay motivated and make it fun!

o Take quality enzymes.

o Rotate your foods to avoid developing allergies as well as maintaining nutritional balance.

o Eat lots of raw organic fruits and vegetables daily.

o Eat organic whole grains, nuts and seeds in moderation.

o Use pure, cold pressed, organic olive oil, or grapeseed oils for salads, <u>moderately</u>.

o Consume a diet rich in Omega 3, 6, and 9 oils.

o Eat 75 percent of your foods in the natural raw state.

o Eat 80 percent alkaline and 20 percent acid foods.

o Thoroughly wash your food with a natural cleanser such as unbuffered Vitamin C crystals or diluted vodka. Rinse well.

o Combine your foods properly.

- Chew your food thoroughly (digestion begins in the mouth).

- Use raw honey, dates, raisins, and stevia for sweeteners.

- Use carob instead of chocolate.

- Flavor your foods with herbs, sea salt or kosher rock salt.

- Limit your dairy products, eating only dairy products from animals fed with organically grown grasses and grains, with no medication administered from birth. Research alternative milk-like drinks gradually eliminating all dairy products (ex: soy, grain or nut milks).

- Eat less meat and only biblically clean meat. Eat meat from animals that have been fed unmedicated, organic grains and grasses only, with a goal toward total elimination of flesh meats.

- Eat your largest meal at breakfast, mid size at lunch and a very light dinner, with a goal of only <u>two</u> meals per day.

- Eat all meals at a regularly scheduled time.

- Have no more than three or four types of food at a meal.

- Grow your own organic foods (if possible).

o Preserve your own foods (dry, freeze, or can).

o Research data on heavy metal and chemical poisoning. Take whatever steps necessary to reduce or eliminate your exposure.

o Reduce electromagnetic fields in your home and office.

o Use cell and portable phones rarely, if at all.

o Strive to make your whole home non-toxic in all ways.

o Remove all amalgam tooth fillings and replace with polyresin fillings.

o Get to bed early and train your body to wake up without an alarm clock.

o Take prescribed drugs **only** when necessary.

o Make short-term and long-term goals and strive for them. Keep a journal.

o Rest one full day each week, preferably Saturday, the Sabbath.

o Meditate/pray each day (and throughout the day).

o Strive to reduce stress. (If you don't, it will kill you!)

o Reduce clutter in your life, house, office, and mind.

- o Spring house clean your office and home. Get rid of anything you do not need. You will be surprised of what ends up in the trash or in the hands of a more needy person.

- o Listen to enjoyable, healing music.

- o Spend time with friends and family.

- o Start a hobby that you enjoy and make time for it in your schedule.

- o Surround yourself with positive and uplifting people.

- o Laugh long and often.

- o Become an Optimist.

- o Help others. Share the information you learn.

- o Be temperate in all things.

- o Simplify, simplify your life!

- o Trust God.

DON'T

- ▪ Use tobacco in any form.

- ▪ Drink alcohol.

- Use drugs.

- Allow decay to pollute the air.

- Get too much sun.

- Wear high heels or narrow toe shoes.

- Apply harmful chemicals to your skin in any form.

- Use harmful cleaning agents or detergents in your home.

- Drink liquids with meals.

- Drink liquids too hot or too cold.

- Drink chlorinated or fluoridated water.

- Eat fruit and vegetables together.

- Eat hydrogenated or partially hydrogenated fats or oils.

- Eat large portions of flesh meats.

- Eat flesh meats treated with antibiotics or fed grain treated with chemicals.

- Eat white bread.

- Eat white flour products (pastries, donuts, pasta, etc.).

- Use sugar or anything made of sugar.

- Use glucose, saccharine, aspartame or olestra.

- Eat fat of meat.

- Eat grease (lard, nucoa).

- Eat foods with preservatives (nitrates, sulfites, and MSG).

- Eat foods too hot or too cold.

- Consume black pepper.

- Consume white distilled vinegar.

- Use aluminum or stainless steel cookware to cook with or eat from (enamel or glass only).

- Consume cottonseed oil in any form.

- Eat too much salt (use small amounts of sea salt when needed).

- Eat before going to bed (at least two hours).

- Drink before going to bed (at least two hours).

- Drink caffeinated beverages (coffee, tea, chocolate, soda).

- Eat between meals.

- Wear footwear with rubber soles (does not allow your body to discharge electrical currents).

- Wear metal under-wired bras.

- Use rubbing alcohol in any form.

- Use OTC (Over-The-Counter) drugs. Try natural remedies instead.

- Use Tampons (chemicals can irritate and cause swelling of vaginal walls).

- Stay up late at night.

- Worry. It will break down your immune system.

- Overwork or under-exercise (hard work never killed anyone, overwork did).

~

"Danger and delight grow on one stick."
- Scottish Proverb

Your Thoughts

29

ENVIRONMENTAL DETOXIFICATION

Check List

The following steps will help eliminate opportunities for toxic growth:

☐ Remove all carpets and install ceramic tile, cork, bamboo or laminated flooring. Hardwood flooring is fine if the finish has been outgased. Carpeting harbors dust and mites, mold, bacteria and other contaminants tracked in from outside, such as lead, asbestos, pesticides and animal feces. If you must have carpeting, the best choices are 100 percent nylon, wool, or cotton. Be sure they are not treated with stain-resistant chemicals, mothproofing, or dyes.

☐ Purchase solid wood furniture and kitchen cabinets instead of pressed wood, particleboard, medium density fiberboard, or plywood, which can all outgas significant levels of toxic formaldehyde over long periods of time.

- ☐ Remove all polyester drapery and replace with 100 percent cotton. Valances are better than curtains as there is less area for the settling of dust.

- ☐ Add indoor houseplants in several rooms. *Lady Palm, Rubber plants, English Ivy and Spider plants* are among the best houseplants to clean the air. Be sure to keep them dusted and not too damp, as mold spores tend to grow.

- ☐ Monitor your home's temperature and humidity. Strive to keep the relative humidity around 40 percent and lower the heat to inhibit the growth of molds, dust mites, bacteria, and viruses.

- ☐ Have your basement evaluated for mold growth and moisture problems. Employ a professional to inspect your home for lead, radon, and asbestos. Have only professionals remove the toxin source.

- ☐ Keep showers wiped down and dry.

- ☐ Do not place damp clothes in the hamper.

- ☐ Ensure that drain spouts are kept clear and carry water away from your home.

- ☐ Monitor windows for moisture accumulation and mold growth.

- ☐ Repair plumbing or roof leeks immediately.

- ☐ Keep one or two feet near the house foundation clear of shrubs and trees.

☐ Maintain air purifiers, dehumidifiers and humidifiers to avoid microbial growth.

☐ Remember, <u>many</u> people do not realize they are sensitive to mold. If you tend to not feel well on rainy and damp days, you may be mold sensitive. See your physician.

☐ Eliminate roaches, lady bugs or any other type of insects in the home. They can cause severe allergic reactions.

☐ Remove all wallpaper (arsenic and mold is found in wallpaper). Paint your rooms with a less toxic paint. Wonderpure by Devoe is less toxic and can be tolerated by most chemically sensitive people.

☐ Cover mattresses and pillows in a high-grade barrier cloth (prevents dust mites from getting into and out of your mattresses and pillows). Use only 100 percent cotton sheets and blankets (preferably organic). Wash bedding weekly in hot water.

☐ Remove as many dust collecting wall hangings and knick-knacks as possible throughout your home.

☐ Remove gas cook stove and install electric.

☐ Remove wood stove. Wood, coal and oil forced air are not healthy ways to heat your home. Hot water or electric baseboards are healthier choices, although they too have dangers.

☐ Install a fire alarm system that doesn't emit radioactive particles into the air and that has a true and proven track record of saving lives. The "Phoenix System 2100" operates with a photoelectric smoke detector and a mechanical heat detector. It is free of any radioactive materials. No outside power source is needed. A must for every home! (see Resource Guide)

☐ Remove all plastic blinds and install metal blinds. When the heat from the sun or your heating system meets with the plastic blinds they emit formaldehyde.

☐ Remove vinyl shower curtains and install tightly woven 100 percent cotton or hemp shower curtains. Vinyls and plastics outgas more VOC's (Volatile Organic Compounds), in the heat and humidity of a shower. After showering, be sure to pull the curtain closed, allowing an opportunity for the curtain to air dry.

☐ Remove all Tupperware and like plastic dishes from your kitchen. They emit formaldehyde. Cook and eat from glass or enamel only.

☐ Do not eat from metal dinnerware (heavy metal will end up in your food and in your body). Use hard plastic dinnerware but do not put them in extremely hot foods, as they will emit chemicals when heated. You may also use porcelain dinnerware, but it may be more difficult to locate. Use wooden spoons for cooking. (Remember to disinfect wooden utensils, as they can hold bacteria.)

☐ Use white distilled vinegar and baking soda for cleaning. Bon Ami can be used for scrubbing tough stains. Keep a spray bottle of equal parts vodka and water in your kitchen and one in your bathroom as a disinfectant. It works great for cleaning up after handling raw meat as well as spraying on the kids' hands before eating. Adding a healthy dose of cayenne pepper to the vodka will deter people from drinking the alcoholic mixture. Use this in place of antibacterial soaps or sprays.

☐ Use baking soda for toothpaste or find toothpaste that does not contain fluoride at your local health store or from companies offering healthier alternatives (see Life Changing Products).

☐ Do not use deodorant. This is usually full of chemicals as well as aluminum, which leach directly into your body. Remember a clean internal and external body doesn't smell. Use apple cider vinegar as an underarm wash. It will kill the bacteria that causes odor.

☐ Do not use hair dyes or perms. The chemicals from these products can be found in the urine within two hours after use. Pure henna is a wonderful hair color and conditioner. Henna has red tones only. You can also use ground black walnut hulls for a darker brown color. Be careful, it stains everything it touches.

☐ Do not use cosmetics, shampoos, conditioners, or soaps you buy at your local grocery or department stores. Most of these products contain harmful chemicals such as sodium laurel sulfate and propylene glycol. Health foods stores will stock safer items for you in some cases. However, even health foods stores stock products that aren't always healthy! Read all labels. I have located a company that has many less toxic, high quality products (see Life Changing Products).

☐ Reduce or eliminate the use of plastic and paper diapers with acrylic gels.

☐ Protect your baby, not the bed. Replace vinyl, plastic and rubber mattress protectors with a naturally waterproof wool pad. Also remember that synthetic foam mattresses, polyester-stuffed toys, bedding and furniture, chemically treated fabrics and draperies, all outgas significant amounts of toxic substances. Also avoid plastic toys and teething rings. Do not store books or magazines in the bedroom as they collect dust and are a breeding ground for mold. Use glass bottles for your baby and do not microwave. Keep children's room as non-toxic as possible!

☐ Do not use plastic food storage bags. They are full of formaldehyde. Do not put food in these bags! Purchase clear cellophane bags made from a wood cellulose fiber. They are available in many sizes (see Resource Guide). Do not use clear plastic wrap to cover food as it too emits dangerous chemicals.

☐ Drink only pure water and lots of it! (Not with meals.) No chlorinated or fluoridated tap water. Make sure you have an adequate whole house filtration system. Remember that chlorine, and other chemicals and metals are absorbed through your skin in the shower. Change filters often!

☐ Remove all footwear at the door. Chemicals, heavy metals, parasites and bacteria can all be tracked into your home from outside. Have slippers available at the door to be worn only indoors.

☐ Do not allow animals in your bedroom. If you are very sick, animals should not be allowed in your home. They are carriers of parasites, which can be very dangerous for an already compromised immune system.

☐ Run high quality air purifiers in all rooms, especially your bedroom. Use an ULPA or HEPA type cleaning device to control particulates, smoke, dust, pollen, and animal dander. Do not use ozone producing devices. Adequate testing has not been done to ensure the safety of these products.

☐ Remove amalgam fillings from your teeth and replace with composite fillings. You may search long and far before you find a dentist that agrees with the dangers of amalgam fillings. Keep searching. The dental trade organizations work closely with dental material manufacturers, therefore, safety concerns are often downplayed. Be sure to ask your dentist what compounds make up the composite fillings. Sometimes, they too have unsafe metals and chemicals added (see Resource Guide).

☐ Maintain good oral hygiene to avoid root canals and crowns. Root canals and crowns are also a source of heavy metal poisoning as well as bacteria that can accumulate in the jawbone. These bacteria can spread throughout the body and cause much havoc.

☐ Do not allow anyone to smoke in your home, office or car.

☐ Air out your home everyday for at least one hour. If you are prone to pollen or mold allergies, run the air cleaner after you have closed the windows to purify the air of incoming particles.

☐ Do not burn incense or scented candles. They are full of chemicals. In fact, some unscented candles also have harmful chemicals and metals in them. It is better not to burn them at all.

☐ Do not wear perfume. If you do, you are making yourself sick as well as everyone around you. There are many lovely smelling essential oils that work wonderfully as perfume. Better yet, use nothing.

☐ Do not use talc or loose powder. It is toxic to breathe, and will be absorbed into the skin.

☐ Use cotton clothing or other natural fibers like linen, hemp or wool. Organic cotton is better but also very expensive. Cotton is one of the most heavily pesticided crops in the United States today. If you choose non-organic cottons, soak the clothing in a solution of vinegar and water for eight hours before wearing them. Dry cleaned clothing is very toxic and should not be worn or be in your home. If you do choose to wear dry cleaned products, ensure that they are hung outside for several hours first and do not store them in your bedroom closet.

☐ Use olive oil, lemon juice and essential oils for furniture polish, not the toxic products you find in the grocery or department stores.

☐ Make your own air fresheners from essential oils. Do not use the toxic brands you can purchase in the grocery or department stores.

☐ Many sunscreens have harmful chemicals. You may purchase a safer product from companies concentrating on healthy alternatives (see Life Changing Products).

☐ Avoid regular exposure to fluorescent lights. The alternative is regular incandescent lighting.

☐ Televisions emit formaldehyde (even when turned off!). If you must have one, have only one and never in the bedroom (smallest screen possible). Sit as far away as possible from the screen.

☐ Do not run electrical cords under your beds or chairs. Unplug all electrical devices when not in use. Avoid sleeping on beds with innersprings, box springs, or metal bed frames. Metal serves as an antenna for electromagnetic fields.

☐ Old computer monitors have extremely high levels of magnetic and electrical radiation. Purchase a low radiation TCO-certified monitor and install a grounded, radiation reducing screen on the monitor. Most of the radiation will be averted away from you.

☐ Limit electrical devices in the bedroom, especially near your head (i.e. electric blanket, clock radio, alarm clocks, etc.). These devices emit electrical and magnetic fields, which can affect the permeability of the barrier surrounding the brain.

☐ Never stand in front of your microwave. Better yet, get rid of it. It kills your food.

☐ As small electrical appliances break, replace them with manual devices (i.e., can opener, mixer). Stand as far away as possible when operating any electrical device.

☐ Electric blow dryers are held close to the head and are dangerous for you as well as damaging your hair. Choose a hairstyle that is more carefree and does not require blow-drying.

☐ Refrigerators and freezers emit harmful Freon which should never be used, much less in our homes. Many companies are now manufacturing these appliances with safer compounds. Research the facts before you buy.

☐ If you live near high voltage power lines, it may be significantly affecting your health. Have an environmental inspection firm check for possible high frequency fields coming from the power lines.

Remember neighbor's homes and electrical grounding practices in your own home are able to significantly increase EMF's as well. If the frequency fields are too high, consider moving. It will be worth the temporary hardship, in order to protect your health and that of your family.

☐ Do not use toxic lawn and garden care products. The long-term health of you and your family should come before the goal of having a perfect lawn or garden. In the real world, weeds and other imperfections are a normal part of nature. Instead of killing the dandelions—eat them.

☐ Do not use harmful insect repellents. If they can peel paint, melt nylon, destroy plastic, wreck wood finishes and damage fishing line, you can only imagine what they are doing to your skin and internal organs.

☐ Keep your home, car and office a place of peace and tranquility. Noise pollution can be as dangerous to our nervous system and health as any other pollution.

☐ Do not keep your vehicle in an attached garage where fumes can enter the house or in a garage under your house. Remember, fumes will rise to the second floor immediately.

☐ When traveling, do not follow closely behind other vehicles, as their fumes will be pulled into the cabin of your vehicle. Keep your ventilation on "recycled air" when in town or following vehicles. Keep it on "fresh air" when traveling in the country, if you aren't allergic to dust, pollen, etc.

☐ Use an air purifier in your car if you are symptomatic after driving in it. Remember that the synthetic materials outgasing in your car, or the air being drawn into the car from the outside, could cause symptoms.

☐ It takes at least two years for a new car to outgas. When you are not driving the car, leave it in the sun with the windows up. The heat will cause it to outgas more quickly. Be sure to open the windows and air well before driving the car. You may also have floor covering and seats ozonated professionally.

☐ Stay away from copy machines or duplicating machines in your office. They are very toxic. Sit as far away as possible or better yet, have them located in an enclosed room with a high quality air purification system.

☐ Fresh air at the office or in school should be a priority on your list. Speak with the building manager to find out the number of air exchanges per hour. More often than not, simply increasing the ventilation within the building cures sick building syndrome. Three things should be considered where air quality is concerned: 1) good ventilation, 2) adequate filtration and 3) hygiene (filters must be kept clean at all times).

☐ Foods! This has been covered in Chapter 4 of this book. However I cannot stress enough the importance of eating whole foods which have had NO chemical processing, as well as eating raw organic foods in their natural state. Remember 80 percent alkaline and 20 percent acid, 75 percent raw and 25 percent cooked.

There are still other ways of improving your health and ridding yourself of diseases. However this list is a great start. Keep alert and research the facts. Once you become aware of all the toxins that can cause illness, you will become an expert as you continue your search for answers.

~

MOTIVATIONAL TIPS

Research the facts! You must do what feels right for you and your family. Keep in mind that because the label says "natural," it doesn't necessarily mean it is healthy for you. A few herbs thrown in with a multitude of chemicals should raise a red flag. Remember health foods stores stock healthy "junk" as well as healthy foods, which means it may be made of more pure ingredients, but is just another version of a salty or sugary junk food.

Do not let this information overwhelm or frighten you. Begin taking gradual steps today to improve your health and that of your family. Stay positive and set short and long-term goals in cleaning up your environment.

Should you have problems in locating any of the alternative products or physicians I have mentioned, please contact me. Additional information is available upon request.

~

"True life is lived when tiny changes occur."

- Leo Tolstoy

CLOSING THOUGHTS

Today, my hope is that each chapter in this book is utilized as a guide to assist you in the quest for information that will lead you to total and vibrant health.

While known diseases and undiagnosed illnesses are on the rise, research rapidly continues, making some information in this book obsolete as I write. Each day brings with it new answers to research studies and new hope for tomorrow. No longer can we continue to mask the symptoms of illness with drugs and/or unnecessary surgeries. Let us continue to educate ourselves and our families, with the vital information we need, to make informed decisions concerning our state of health and the methods we choose to treat our illnesses.

If illness hasn't struck you personally, it most assuredly has touched the lives of family or friends. Do you not owe it to yourself and your loved ones to be as healthy as you can be? You deserve good health. You can have good health. However, it comes with a price. That price is dedication and discipline to obeying the health laws within these pages. Your ongoing wellness will demand your vigilant and continuing research to protect yourself and your family from the environmental toxins you are bombarded with each and every day.

How long will we...

⇒ prescribe mind-altering drugs to our over active children? Until we realize that food allergies and environmental toxins are the culprits in most cases.

⇒ demand antibiotics from our physicians for every ailment? Until we realize that drugs break down the immune system and that many illnesses can be successfully treated with natural remedies.

⇒ tolerate continuous sleep deprivation? Until stress, emotional problems, allergies and nutritional deficiencies are identified and controlled.

⇒ work day after day with no rest and relaxation? Until we are hospitalized with some dreaded condition such as heart failure or stroke.

⇒ carry around an extra fifty pounds of body fat accompanied by insatiable hunger? Until we start eating foods that nourish the body and practicing self-control.

⇒ experience fatigue, disease, pain and suffering? Until the laws of health are followed and healthy lifestyle changes are implemented.

⇒ live and work in environmental pollution, allowing the demise of our immune system? Until we educate ourselves of the harmful side effects of chemicals, radiation, heavy metals, and electromagnetic fields and reduce or eliminate them.

⇒ remain depressed, lonely and hopeless? Until we ask God to change us and trust that he will.

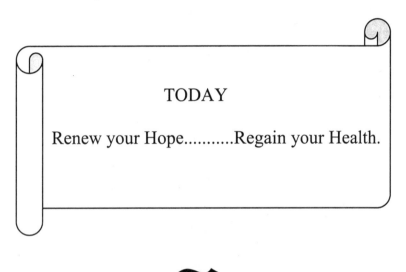

TODAY

Renew your Hope...........Regain your Health.

"An investment in knowledge pays the best interest."

- Benjamin Franklin

The Answer

I prayed for courage
He sent a danger
And I became brave.

I prayed for wisdom
He gave me a problem
And I grew wise.

I prayed for strength
He sent me a weakness
And I grew strong.

I prayed for faith
He handed me doubts
And I learned to trust.

I prayed for love
He sent a child
And I became lovable.

by Ralph W. Seager

"You cannot read this article merely one time and truly obtain and appreciate the magnitude of its content. Read it slowly, line by line, thought by thought…. Read it often."
— Brenda O. Brown

THE GOD MEMORANDUM

(Excerpt from his book entitled *The Greatest Miracle in the World*— pages 99-115.)

by Og Mandino

Take counsel, I hear your cry. It passes through the darkness, filters through the clouds, mingles with starlight, and finds its way to my heart on the path of a sunbeam. I have anguished over the cry of a hare choked in the noose of a snare, a sparrow tumbled from the nest of its mother, a child thrashing helplessly in a pond, and a son shedding his blood on a cross. Know that I hear you, also. Be at peace. **Be calm.**

I bring thee relief for your sorrow for I know its cause... And its cure. You weep for all your childhood dreams that have vanished with the years. You weep for all your self-esteem that has been corrupted by failure. You weep for all your potential that has been bartered for security. You weep for all your individuality that has been trampled by mobs. You weep for all your talent that has been wasted through misuse.

You look upon yourself with disgrace and you turn in terror from the image you see in the pool. Who is this mockery of humanity staring back at you with bloodless eyes of shame? Where is the grace of your manner, the beauty of your figure, the quickness of your movement, the clarity of your mind, the brilliance of your tongue? Who stole your goods? Is the thief's identity known to you, as it is to me?

Once you placed your head in a pillow of grass in your father's field and looked up at a cathedral of clouds and knew that all the gold of Babylon would be yours in time. Once you read from many books and wrote on many tablets, convinced beyond any doubt that all the wisdom of Solomon would be equaled and surpassed by you. And the seasons would flow into years until lo, you would reign supreme in your own garden of Eden.

Dost thou remember who implanted those plans and dreams and seeds of hope within you? You cannot. You have no memory of that moment when first you emerged from your mother's womb and I placed my hand on your soft brow. And the secret I whispered in your small ear when I bestowed my blessings upon you?

Remember our secret? You cannot. The passing years have destroyed your recollection, for they have filled your mind with fear and doubt and anxiety and remorse and hate and there is no room for joyful memories where these beasts habitate. Weep no more. I am with you ... and this moment is the dividing line of your life. All that has gone before is like unto no more than that time you slept within your mother's womb. What is past is dead. Let the dead bury the dead.

This day you return from the living dead. This day, like unto Elijah with the widow's son, I stretch myself upon thee three times and you live again. This day, like unto Elisha with the Shunammite's son, I put my mouth upon your mouth and my eyes upon your eyes and my hands upon your hands and your flesh is warm again.

This day, like unto Jesus at the tomb of Lazarus, I command you to come forth and you will walk from your cave of doom to begin a new life. This is your birthday. This is your new date of birth. Your first life, like unto a play of the theatre, was only a rehearsal. This time the curtain is up. This time the world watches and waits to applaud. This time you will not fail!

Light your candles. Share your cake. Pour the wine. You have been reborn. Like a butterfly from its chrysalis you will fly ... fly as high as you wish, and neither the wasps nor dragonflies nor mantids of mankind shall obstruct your mission or your search for the true riches of life. Feel my hand upon thy head. Attend to my wisdom. Let me share with you, again, the secret you heard at your birth and forgot. You are my greatest miracle. You are the greatest miracle in the world. Those were the first words you ever heard. Then you cried. They all cry ...

You did not believe me then ... and nothing has happened in the intervening years to correct your disbelief. For how could you be a miracle when you consider yourself a failure at the most menial of tasks? How can you be a miracle when you have little confidence in dealing with the most trivial of responsibilities? How can you be a miracle when you are shackled by debt and lie awake in torment over whence will come tomorrow's bread?

Enough. The milk that is spilled is sour. Yet, how many prophets, how many wise men, how many poets, how many artists, how many composers, how many scientists, how many philosophers and messengers have I sent with word of your divinity, your potential for godliness, and the secrets of achievement? How did you treat them?

Still I love you and I am with you now, through these words, to fulfill the prophet who announced that the Lord shall set his hand again, the second time, to recover the remnant of his people. I have set my hand again. This is the second time. You are my remnant. It is of no avail to ask, haven't you known, haven't you heard, hasn't it been told to you from the beginning; haven't you understood from the foundations of the earth? You have not known; you have not heard; you have not understood. You have been told that you are a divinity in disguise, a god playing a fool.

You have been told that you are a special piece of work, noble in reason, infinite in faculties, express and admirable in form and moving, like an angel in action, like a god in apprehension. You have been told that you are the salt of the earth. You were given the secret even of moving mountains, of performing the impossible. You believed no one. You burned your map to happiness, you abandoned your claim to peace of mind, you snuffed out the candles that had been placed along your destined path of glory, and then you stumbled, lost and frightened, in the darkness of futility and self-pity, until you fell into a hell of your own creation.

Then you cried and beat your breast and cursed the luck that had befallen you. You refused to accept the consequences of your own petty thoughts and lazy deeds and you searched for a scapegoat on which to blame your failure. How quickly you found one. You blamed me! You cried that your handicaps, your mediocrity, your lack of opportunity, your failures ... were the will of God! **You were wrong!**

Let us take inventory. Let us, first, call a roll of your handicaps. For how can I ask you to build a new life lest you have the tools? Are you blind? Does the sun rise and fall without your witness? No. You can see ... **and the hundred million receptors I have placed in your eyes** enable you to enjoy the magic of a leaf, a snowflake, a pond, an eagle, a child, a cloud, a star, a rose, a rainbow ... and the look of love. *Count one blessing.*

Are you deaf? Can a baby laugh or cry without your attention? No. You can hear ... **and the twenty-four thousand fibers I have built in each of your ears** vibrate to the wind in the trees, the tides on the rocks, the majesty of an opera, a robin's plea, children at play ... and the words I love you. *Count another blessing.*

Are you mute? Do your lips move and bring forth only spittle? No. You can speak ... as can no other of my creatures, and your words can calm the angry, uplift the despondent, goad the quitter, cheer the unhappy, warm the lonely, praise the worthy, encourage the defeated, teach the ignorant... and say I love you. *Count another blessing.*

Are you paralyzed? Does your helpless form despoil the land? No. You can move. You are not a tree condemned to a small plot while the wind and world abuses you. You can stretch and run and dance and work, **for within you I have designed five hundred muscles, two hundred bones, and seven miles of nerve fibre all synchronized by me to do your bidding.** *Count another blessing.*

Are you unloved and unloving? Does loneliness engulf you, night and day? No. No more. For now you know love's secret, that to receive love it must be given with no thought of its return. To love for fulfillment, satisfaction, or pride is no love. Love is a gift on which no return is demanded. Now you know that to love unselfishly is its own reward. And even should love not be returned it is not lost, for love not reciprocated will flow back to you and soften and purify your heart. *Count another blessing. Count twice.*

Is your heart stricken? Does it leak and strain to maintain your life? No. **Your heart is strong. Touch your chest and feel its rhythm, pulsating, hour after hour, day and night, thirty-six million beats each year, year after year, asleep or awake,** pumping your blood through more than sixty thousand miles of veins, arteries, and tubing... pumping more than six hundred thousand gallons each year. Man has never created such a machine. *Count another blessing.*

Are you diseased of skin? Do people turn in horror when you approach? No. Your skin is clear and a marvel of creation, needing only that you tend it with soap and oil and brush and care. In time all steels will tarnish and rust, but not your skin. Eventually the strongest of metals will wear, with use, but not that layer that I have constructed around you. Constantly it renews itself, old cells replaced by new, just as the old you is now replaced by the new. *Count another blessing.*

Are your lungs befouled? Does your breath of life struggle to enter your body? No. Your portholes to life support you even in the vilest of environments of your own making, and **they labor always to filter life-giving oxygen through six hundred million pockets of folded flesh while they rid your body of gaseous wastes.** *Count another blessing.*

Is your blood poisoned? Is it diluted with water and pus? No. **Within your five quarts of blood are twenty-two trillion blood cells and within each cell are millions of molecules and within each molecule is an atom oscillating at more than ten million times each second. Each second, two million of your blood cells die to be replaced by two million more in a resurrection that has continued since your first birth.** As it has always been inside, so now it is on your outside. *Count another blessing.*

Are you feeble of mind? Can you no longer think for yourself? No. **Your brain is the most complex structure in the universe. I know. Within its three pounds are thirteen billion nerve cells, more than three times as many cells as there are people on your earth. To help you file away every perception, every sound, every taste, every smell, every action you have experienced since the day of your birth, I have implanted, within your cells, more than one thousand billion billion protein molecules.**

Every incident in your life is there waiting only your recall. And, **to assist your brain in the control of your body I have dispersed, throughout your form, four million pain-sensitive structures, five hundred thousand touch detectors, and more than two hundred thousand temperature detectors.** No nation's gold is better protected than you. None of your ancient wonders are greater than you.

You are my finest creation. **Within you is enough atomic energy to destroy any of the world's great cities... and rebuild it.** Are you poor? Is there no gold or silver in your purse? No. You are rich! Together we have just counted your wealth. Study the list. *Count them again. Tally your assets!*

Why have you betrayed yourself? Why have you cried that all the blessings of humanity were removed from you? Why did you deceive yourself that you were powerless to change your life? Are you without talent, senses, abilities, pleasures, instincts, sensations, and pride? Are you without hope? Why do you cringe in the shadows, a giant defeated, awaiting only sympathetic transport into the welcome void and dampness of hell?

You have so much. Your blessings overflow your cup ... and you have been unmindful of them, like a child spoiled in luxury, since I have bestowed them upon you with generosity and regularity. Answer me. Answer yourself.

What rich man, old and sick, feeble and helpless, would not exchange all the gold in his vault for the blessings you have treated so lightly? Know then the first secret to happiness and success - that you possess, even now, every blessing necessary to achieve great glory. They are your treasure, your tools with which to build, starting today, the foundation for a new and better life.

Therefore, I say unto you, _**count your blessings**_ and know that you already are my greatest creation. **This is the first law** you must obey in order to perform the greatest miracle in the world, the return of your humanity from living death.

And be grateful for your lessons learned in poverty. For he is not poor who has little; only he that desires much ... and true security lies not in the things one has but in the things one can do without. Where are the handicaps that produced your failure? They existed only in your mind. Count your blessings.

And the second law is like unto the first. _**Proclaim your rarity.**_ You had condemned yourself to a potter's field, and there you lay, unable to forgive your own failure, destroying yourself with self-hate, self-incrimination, and revulsion at your crimes against yourself and others. Are you not perplexed? Do you not wonder why I am able to forgive your failures, your transgressions, your pitiful demeanor ... when you cannot forgive yourself?

I address you now, for three reasons. You need me. You are not one of a herd heading for destruction in a gray mass of mediocrity. And ... you are a great rarity. Consider a painting by Rembrant or a bronze by Degas or a violin by Stradivarius or a play by Shakespeare. They have great value for two reasons: their creators were masters and they are few in number. Yet there are more than one of each of these.

On that reasoning you are the most valuable treasure on the face of the earth, for you know who created you and there is only one of you. Never, in all the seventy billion humans who have walked this planet since the beginning of time has there been anyone exactly like you. Never, until the end of time, will there be another such as you. You have shown no knowledge or appreciation of your uniqueness. Yet, you are the rarest thing in the world. From your father, in his moment of supreme love, flowed countless seeds of love, more than four hundred million in number. All of them, as they swam within your mother, gave up the ghost and died. All except one! You.

You alone persevered within the loving warmth of your mother's body, searching for your other half, a single cell from your mother so small that more than two million would be necessary to fill an acorn shell. Yet, despite impossible odds, in that vast ocean of darkness and disaster, you persevered, found that infinitesimal cell, joined with it, and began a new life. **Your life**.

You arrived, bringing with you, as does every child, the message that I was not yet discouraged of man. Two cells now united in a miracle. **Two cells, each containing twenty-three chromosomes and within each chromosome hundreds of genes**, which would govern every characteristic about you, from the color of your eyes to the charm of your manner, to the size of your brain.

With all the combinations at my command, beginning with that single sperm from your father's four hundred million, through the hundreds of genes in each of the chromosomes from your mother and father, I could have created three hundred thousand billion humans, each different from the other. But who did I bring forth? You! One of a kind. Rarest of the rare. A priceless treasure, possessed of qualities in mind and speech and movement and appearance and actions as no other who has ever lived, lives, or shall live.

Why have you valued yourself in pennies when you are worth a king's ransom? Why did you listen to those who demeaned you ... and far worse, why did you believe them? Take counsel. No longer hide your rarity in the dark. Bring it forth. Show the world. Strive not to walk as your brother walks, nor talk as your leader

246 DYING IN THE LAND OF PLENTY

talks, nor labor as do the mediocre. Never do as another. Never imitate. For how do you know that you may not imitate evil; and he who imitates evil always goes beyond the example set, while he who imitates what is good always falls short. Imitate no one. Be yourself. Show your rarity to the world and they will shower you with gold.

This then is the second law. *Proclaim your rarity*. And now you have received two laws. **Count your blessings**! **Proclaim your rarity**!

You have no handicaps. You are not mediocre. You nod. You force a smile. You admit your self-deception. What of your next complaint? Opportunity never seeks thee? Take counsel and it shall come to pass, for now I give you the law of success in every venture. Many centuries ago this law was given to your forefathers from a mountaintop. Some heeded the law and lo, their life was filled with the fruit of happiness, accomplishment, gold, and peace of mind.

Most listened not, for they sought magic means, devious routes, or waited for the devil called luck to deliver to them the riches of life. They waited in vain ... just as you waited, and then they wept, blaming their lack of fortune.

The law is simple. Young or old, pauper or king, white or black, male or female ... all can use the secret to their advantage; for all the rules and speeches and scriptures of success and how to attain it, only one method has never failed ... **whomsoever shall compel ye to go with him one mile ... go with him two. This then is the third law** ... the secret that will produce riches and acclaim beyond your dreams. **Go another mile!**

The only certain means of success is to render more and better service than is expected of you, no matter what your task may be. This is a habit followed by all successful people since the beginning of time. Therefore I saith the surest way to doom yourself to mediocrity is to perform only the work for which you are paid.

Think not ye are being cheated if you deliver more than the silver you receive. For there is a pendulum to all life and the sweat you deliver, if not rewarded today, will swing back tomorrow, tenfold. The mediocre never goes another mile, for why should he cheat himself, he thinks. But you are not mediocre. To go another mile is a privilege you must appropriate by your own initiative. You cannot, you must not avoid it. Neglect it, do only as little as the others, and the responsibility for your failure is yours alone.

You can no more render service without receiving just compensation than you can withhold the rendering of it without suffering the loss of reward. Cause and effect, means and ends, seed and fruit, these cannot be separated. The effect already blooms in the cause, the end pre-exists in the means, and the fruit is always in the seed. **Go another mile**.

Concern yourself not, should you serve an ungrateful master. Serve him more. And instead of him, let it be me who is in your debt, for then you will know that every minute, every stroke of extra service will be repaid. And worry not, should your reward not come soon. For the longer payment is withheld, the better for you ... and compound interest on compound interest is this law's greatest benefit.

You cannot command success, you can only deserve it ... and now you know the great secret necessary in order to merit its rare reward. **Go another mile!**

Where is this field whence you cried there was no opportunity? Look! Look around thee. See, where only yesterday you wallowed on the refuse of self-pity, you now walk tall on a carpet of gold. Nothing has changed... except you, but you are everything.

You are my greatest miracle. You are the greatest miracle in the world. *And now the laws of happiness and success are three.*

<u>Count your blessings</u>! <u>Proclaim your rarity</u>! <u>Go another mile</u>!

Be patient with your progress. To count your blessings with gratitude, to proclaim your rarity with pride, to go an extra mile and then another, these acts are not accomplished in the blinking of an eye. Yet, that which you acquire with most difficulty you retain the longest; as those who have earned a fortune are more careful of it than those by whom it was inherited.

And fear not as you enter your new life. Every noble acquisition is attended with its risks. He who fears to encounter the one must not expect to obtain the other. Now you know you are a miracle. And there is no fear in a miracle.

Be proud. You are not the momentary whim of a careless creator experimenting in the laboratory of life. You are not a slave of forces that you cannot comprehend. You are a free manifestation of no force but mine, of no love but mine. You were made with a purpose. Feel my hand. Hear my words. You need me ... and I need you. We have a world to rebuild ... and if it requireth a miracle what is that to us? We are both miracles and now we have each other.

Never have I lost faith in you since that day when I first spun you from a giant wave and tossed you helplessly on the sands. As you measure time that was more than five hundred million years ago. There were many models, many shapes, many sizes, before I reached perfection in you more than thirty thousand years ago. I have made no further effort to improve on you in all these years.

For how could one improve on a miracle? You were a marvel to behold and I was pleased. I gave you this world and dominion over it. Then, to enable you to reach your full potential I placed my hand upon you, once more, and endowed you with powers unknown to any other creature in the universe, even unto this day.

I gave you the power to think. I gave you the power to love.
I gave you the power to will. I gave you the power to laugh.
I gave you the power to imagine. I gave you the power to create.
I gave you the power to plan. I gave you the power to speak.
I gave you the power to pray. I gave you the power to heal.

My pride in you knew no bounds. You were my ultimate creation, my greatest miracle. A complete living being. One who can adjust to any climate, any hardship, any challenge. One who can manage his own destiny without any interference from me. One who can translate a sensation or perception, not by instinct, but by thought and deliberation into whatever action is best for himself and all humanity.

Thus we come to the fourth law of success and happiness ... for I gave you one more power, a power so great that not even my angels possess it. I gave you ... **the power to choose.**

With this gift I placed you even above my angels ... for angels are not free to choose sin. I gave you complete control over your destiny. I told you to determine, for yourself, your own nature in accordance with your own free will. Neither heavenly nor earthly in nature, you were free to fashion yourself in whatever form you preferred. You had the power to choose to degenerate into the lowest forms of life, but you also had the power, out of your soul's judgment, to be reborn into the higher forms, which are divine. I have never withdrawn your great power, **the power to choose.**

What have you done with this tremendous force? Look at yourself. Think of the choices you have made in your life and recall, now, those bitter moments when you would fall to your knees if only you had the opportunity to choose again. What is past is past ... and now you know the fourth great law of happiness and success ... **Use wisely, your power of choice.**

Choose to love ... rather than hate. Choose to laugh ... rather than cry.

Choose to create ... rather than destroy. Choose to persevere ... rather than quit.

Choose to praise ... rather than gossip. Choose to heal ... rather than wound.

Choose to give ... rather than steal. Choose to act ... rather than procrastinate.

Choose to grow ... rather than rot. Choose to pray ... rather than curse.

Choose to live ... rather than die.

Now you know that your misfortunes were not my will, for all power was vested in you, and the accumulation of deeds and thoughts which placed you on the refuse of humanity were your doing, not mine. My gifts of power were too large for your small nature. Now you have grown tall and wise and the fruits of the land will be yours.

You are more than a human being, you are a human becoming.

You are capable of great wonders. Your potential is unlimited. Who else, among my creatures, has mastered fire? Who else, among my creatures, has conquered gravity, has pierced the heavens, has conquered disease and pestilence and drought?

Never demean yourself again! Never settle for the crumbs of life! Never hide your talents, from this day hence!

Remember the child who says, "when I am a big boy." But what is that? For the big boy says. "when I grow up." And then the grown up, he says, "when I am wed." But to be wed, what is that, after all? The thought then changes to "when I retire." And then, retirement comes, and he looks back over it and somehow he has missed it all and it is gone. Enjoy this day, today ... and tomorrow, tomorrow.

You have performed the greatest miracle in the world. You have returned from a living death. You will feel self-pity no more and each new day will be a challenge and a joy. You have been born again ... but just as before, you can choose failure and despair or success and happiness. The choice is yours. The choice is exclusively yours. I can only watch, as before ... in pride ... or sorrow.

Remember, then, the four laws of happiness and success.
Count your blessings.
Proclaim your rarity.
Go another mile.
Use wisely your power of choice.
And one more, to fulfill the other four. Do all things with love
... love for yourself, love for all others, and love for me.

Wipe away your tears. Reach out, grasp my hand, and stand straight. Let me cut the grave cloths that have bound you. This day you have been notified.

YOU ARE THE GREATEST MIRACLE IN THE WORLD!

~

"Beloved, I wish above all things that thou may prosper and be in health."
- 3 John 2

LIFE CHANGING PRODUCTS

In a perfect world, we would obtain all the nutrients our bodies need from the foods we consume. Unfortunately, polluted air and water, depleted soil and the fast-food, fast-paced world we live in today makes this virtually impossible. Therefore most people need additional support from quality supplements derived from natural sources to obtain the vibrant health they desire.

Rigidly following the protocol outlined in this book, I actually discovered very few truly "Life Changing Products." I consumed hundreds of different supplements and products in an effort to recover my health. Many products and supplements were ineffective as well as expensive and proved to do very little if anything for my chronic state of health.

Our bodies need to be in a <u>constant</u> cleansing and rebuilding mode. The formulas, which I discovered and which actually assisted in turning my health around and continues to maintain my health today, are briefly explained below. Not all people will need to take the drastic measures I did to regain their health. However, if you do not start now you will without a doubt be facing the same situation in your lifetime. Disease and chronic illness have many names. Today's illnesses are being branded with new names on an all too frequent basis. Don't be another statistic. Our website has more detailed information as well as links to the companies that manufacture or distribute these products.

Once I began the cleansing and rebuilding process, I felt worse and experienced additional symptoms. Concerned that possibly I was allergic to the products or some other foreign substance I sought my doctor for advice.

"Herxheimer Reaction" also referred to as a "healing crisis" is nothing more than a sign that your body is eliminating toxins. I developed rashes I had never experienced before, had pain in areas that I had never had pain before. These symptoms occur as the body cleanses and repairs itself. The discomfort is usually short and mild. If this reaction becomes more severe, check with your physician. The doctor may decrease or change the protocol somewhat, allowing the detoxification process to take place more gradually.

Before we can begin to rebuild our bodies we must begin the cleansing process. Our blood, lymph system, vital organs, digestive tract, skin, etc. all need to be targeted in the cleansing process. **Happy Colon** addresses the intestinal tract. **Livatone** and **Livatone Plus** address the liver and all its multi-functions. **Go-Way** will attack parasitic problems, eradicating them, leaving the intestinal tract able to absorb the nutrients it so desperately needs to thrive. **Sun Chlorella** will assist in carrying heavy metals and toxic chemicals out of the body as well as begin rebuilding the body with concentrated amounts of chlorophyll.

Once my body was mid-stream in the cleansing process, it was necessary to replace the beneficial bacteria, or flora in my digestive tract. Our modern lifestyle, which includes antibiotic drug use, chlorinated water, chemical ingestion, pollution and poor diet, is responsible for eradicating much of the beneficial bacteria in our bodies. A lack of beneficial microbes often results in poor intestinal and immune system health, contributing to a wide range of symptoms and illnesses. **Primal Defense** is a probiotic that is virtually unharmed by the stomach acid and is not temperature sensitive, thus making it a much more potent and effective product than most probiotics on the store shelf today.

To bring my state of health to its optimum level some very potent compounds were needed, that were able to combat viruses, bacteria, fungi, and infections. The **Beta-1, 3-D Glucan** detailed below is a superior product bringing life-changing results in the overall health of my body. **Oil of Oregano** and **Oregacyn** are also great immune builders and should be found in every home.

As I continued to cleanse and rebuild it was necessary that I consume a potent, balanced, easily absorbable source of vitamins and minerals. The soil our food is grown in, is depleted of valuable nutrients, the delivery time from the garden to our table can take weeks, the processes used to prepare our food, leave our meals virtually empty of vital nutrients. In today's world we can no longer obtain the necessary nutrients in the amounts needed from our foods. **Seasilver** resolves this problem by providing a very potent, highly absorbable liquid supplement that can be safely taken on a daily basis. Realizing that many enzymes are lost in the foods we eat for many various factors, most people are in need of a high potency and balanced enzyme supplement. **OmegaZyme** is just that!

Of course I needed to also consider the exterior cleansing of my body. **Exfoliating gloves** will make each and every shower an exhilarating event, never before experienced with a wash cloth or sponge.

As I externally cleansed my body, hair, and teeth with **personal care products** that I knew were toxic and were proven dangerous, I continued my search for healthier alternatives. It served no purpose for me to cleanse internally, rebuild and then externally apply toxic chemicals that were absorbed back into my body. My search ended with a company that truly had my health in mind.

Visit our website at (www.marpesolutions.com) for more detailed information on all of the products listed. You may purchase any of these products and supplements directly through our website. Various companies manufacture these products. It would have been very convenient to find all these quality products within one company. Traveling that route was extremely disappointing for me. Not all supplements are the same. That is what makes these products unique. The individual companies specialize in their own particular product and processes.

You may also contact me via email at: (marpesolutions@ascent.net) or mail correspondence directly to me at: Marpe´ Solutions, 523 Granville Hill Rd, Sherburne, New York 13460. I will be glad to assist you or put you in contact with the manufacturers and highly trained staff of these products.

A quarterly newsletter bringing you the latest research results, health tips and new services and products is being developed and will be released later this year. Stay in touch!

¤¤¤

Below is a brief description of our "Life Changing Products"

<u>Happy Colon</u>

That's right, Happy Colon, and that is what I achieved after cleansing with this formula.

When we fail to follow the health laws outlined in this book, it is inevitable that the digestive system will suffer. Most people in the United States are walking around in a constipated state. We should have a bowel elimination for every meal we eat. If we do not, the foods in our intestinal tract begin to ferment and putrefy, causing poisons to be absorbed into our blood stream, ultimately poisoning all organs in the body. Constipation doesn't kill you immediately, but as toxins build up, your whole body is more susceptible to disease. Joint problems, headaches, skin disorders, a "sick all over" and run-down feeling are common signs of constipation.

As layers and layers of corrosion begin to build up on the intestinal walls, the sides of the colon become so hard the peristaltic muscle cannot function properly. We then resort to straining, which eventually leads to hemorrhoids. Many people become dependent on enemas, which is very dangerous. We are training our body to perform its normal functions by this artificial means of elimination.

This product is one of the very best, all natural colon cleansers I have found and is reasonably priced.

Go-Way

As discussed earlier in this book, parasites are a growing problem in the American people today. They rob us from desperately needed nutrients, leaving their waste products behind to further poison our systems. Because the symptoms of parasitic infection closely resemble many other digestive problems, they go unnoticed and untreated. After all, it is very difficult to imagine or admit that we may have living creatures crawling around in our bodies. This product is safe and effective and very reasonably priced.

Livatone and Livatone Plus

The liver cleanses the body of all the poisons that infiltrate it daily, including fat; cholesterol, alcohol, drugs, artificial colors, flavors, and preservatives, airborne pollutants; and poisons in water and food. Since all the toxins we take in each day must be filtered through the liver, it is extremely important that we concentrate on cleansing and rebuilding the liver immediately.

Livatone is a natural liver tonic containing the liver herbs St. Mary's Thistle, Globe artichoke and Dandelion, combined with the amino acid taurine, and lecithin. It also contains natural sources of chlorophyll, carotenoids and fiber and is a great product for anyone wanting to generally improve the function of his or her liver.

This company produces an even more powerful formula for metabolic problems or dysfunction's of the liver, called Livatone Plus. The product contains the liver herb St. Mary's Thistle, combined with sulfur bearing amino acids taurine, glycine, cysteine and glutamine. Livatone Plus also contains all the important B vitamins and lipotrophic cofactors such as inositol, folic acid and biotin. It contains antioxidants to reduce liver damage and inflammation, such as Green Tea, Vitamins C, E and natural beta-carotene. Lecithin and broccoli powder have also been added to help the liver function.

As stated earlier in my book, during my extreme illness, my liver was not functioning properly at all. Nothing my doctor or I tried seemed to work. The medical profession was at a loss. When I combined the protocol that I have outlined in this book as well as taking this powerful supplement, my liver function improved greatly and continues to function normally today. Dr. Sandra Cabot, the developer of this great product has also authored an easy to read, easy to understand book entitled "The Liver Cleansing Diet" to assist in the liver cleansing and rebuilding process. A real eye opener! You will never view your liver the same again after reading this book.

Sun Chlorella

Chlorella is a green, single-cell fresh-water algae with a host of nutrients. Each chlorella cell is a self-sufficient organism with all of the plant's life functions taking place inside the cell. The result is an unusually high concentration of important nutrients in the chlorella plant.

Chlorella has more than 20 different vitamins and minerals and provides an abundance of naturally occurring beta-carotene, which has been said to effectively assist the body to combat UV radiation damage to the skin and the stress of pollutants on the lungs. This plant is 50 to 60 percent protein and is one of the highest natural sources of DNA and RNA. Chlorella is one of the highest natural sources of chlorophyll and contains iron, iodine and zinc. It is also rich in lysine, which is often lacking in our high-wheat diets. Finally, chlorella contains more Vitamin B-12 than beef liver.

My doctor advised me to take chlorella while I was undergoing chelation treatments for the removal of heavy metals. I also put my son on the same chlorella treatment as he too experienced many of the symptoms of toxicity that I did. Carrying my child for nine months in a toxic body brought forth a toxic child as well.

Again, researching the quality of the supplements I was taking, lead me to realize that the chlorella I was consuming was not being absorbed readily into my body due to the fact that the cell walls of the plant were not broken. Further research enlightened me to the fact that even some brands that claim to have broken cell chlorella used heat-treated methods and chemicals which were not effective in breaking the cell walls. Many of the important nutrients were damaged resulting in an inferior product.

*Eventually I located a product that uses a special patented process that breaks the cell wall naturally. This product is called **Sun Chlorella.** The best of the best! Testimonials of customers who have used various chlorella products have experienced outstanding results from this product.*

Beta-1, 3-D Glucan

The immune response is the body's way of defending itself against foreign substances that invade it. These invaders, like viruses, bacteria, fungi, etc., cause infection and disease.

Beta-1, 3-D Glucan is a highly purified, unique compound that is extracted from the cell walls of common baker's yeast and does not contain yeast proteins that could cause an allergic reaction. It is completely safe and has no known toxic properties or adverse side effects. This product is truly a breakthrough in preventative nutrition.

Beta-1, 3-D Glucan works by activating the immune cells known as macrophages. These macrophages trap and consume foreign substances in the body. It is a powerful antioxidant, a natural radioprotective compound, assists substances like antibiotics, antifungals, antiparasitics and cholesterol reducing drugs, to work better in the body. It helps to maintain joint health and aids in tissue repair and regeneration. However the most important effect it has on the body is the anti-neoplastic effect, making the macrophages recognize and destroy mutated cells.

Everyone can benefit from this product, including any person with impaired immunity from any cause such as infectious diseases, HIV, radiation or chemotherapy patients and aging or geriatric patients. People who are in a chronic state of illness or who have diabetes may greatly benefit from this product. Persons exposed to prolonged radiation from external sources such as UV rays or EMF's will benefit as this supplement helps create a radioprotective effect. Those individuals who have a high risk of cardiovascular disease, poor nutrition, physical or emotional stress or work out extensively may experience improved health as well. Even for the healthiest person, Beta-1, 3-D Glucan can be a key instrument in maintaining one's health.

This product has been researched and documented by some of the most prestigious universities in the world.

Beware of copycat products with unduly high levels of proteins, fats and other contaminants. Do not expose yourself to the allergenic compounds found in semi-purified products. Scientific tests have proven that this brand of Beta-1, 3-D Glucan is the best in <u>any</u> and <u>every</u> category that counts!

In my lengthy search for supplements that were able to truly assist in turning my immune system around, I was led to the discovery of Beta Glucan. Testing several different brand names for no less than a three-month period for each brand, I noticed very few beneficial properties. It was not until I located this particular brand of Beta-1, 3-D Glucan did I see a remarkable difference. There truly is no better Beta Glucan. The manufacturer of this product will provide you information on their extensive and costly processes in manufacturing this amazing product as well as documented test results of the top five Beta Glucan products on the market today. I am confident once you experience this Beta Glucan, your search will be over. Also ask about the famous Formula III lotion which contains Beta-1, 3-D Glucan. It is a one-of-a-kind healing lotion when intense treatment is needed.

The manufacturer of this product maintains a highly trained and experienced staff of doctors and specialists who are always available to answer your questions.

<u>Oil of Oregano/Oregacyn</u>

Oregano! We use it in lots of dishes but did you realize how good it is for you? Just adding oregano to our food has healing benefits. However, pure oil of oregano is an extraordinary product. Although there are a wide variety of plants that are confused with oregano, including marjoram, thyme and sage, true oregano grows wild in Mediterranean regions such as Greece. Dr. Cass Ingram, D.O., has written a book entitled *The Cure is in the*

Cupboard, in which he unveils the health benefits of oregano and oil of oregano. He notes that "wild oregano is a veritable natural mineral treasure-house, containing a density of minerals that would rival virtually any food." Wild oregano is rich in many minerals that include calcium, magnesium, zinc, iron, potassium, copper, boron, and manganese. Vitamins C and A (beta carotene) and niacin also are present in oregano.

These products have many useful purposes. They are used to halt the growth of microbes in foods, treats internal and external fungi and yeasts as well as skin conditions such as psoriasis and eczema. They are also effective against bacteria and parasites and contain anti-allergy properties. Dr. Ingram notes, oregano is "one of the world's finest natural medicines, that is if it's true oregano."

Pure Oil of Oregano and Oregacyn are staples in my home. I reach for them every time we experience colds, coughs, bronchitis, sore throats, etc. They also work well for me in assisting the control of candidiasis. The oil is used for many ailments. I would challenge you to research further into this powerful herb and use it in improving the health of your family. Dr. Ingram's books as well as true Oil of Oregano and Oregacyn are available on our website. Don't miss this great reading. Once you realize the benefits of oregano, your home will never be without it.

Seasilver

A 100 percent whole food (plant-based) nutritional supplement with proprietary ingredients and proprietary processing techniques. This product works in perfect harmony with Mother Nature by observing all health laws, guaranteeing all nutrients will be absorbed at the cellular level.

For over 25 years worldwide, every Medical Doctor, Osteopath, Chiropractor and Naturopathic Physicians agree that we must do seven basic things (Balance, Cleanse, Purify, Nourish, Oxygenate, Protect, and Strengthen) to have optimum health. We live in a world that has environmental problems, from the air we breathe to the water we drink. Our foods today are becoming more and more depleted of vital nutrients because of depleted soils, chemical fertilization and improper food preparation. Combined with the stress of everyday life from society, family, career, and financial challenges, our need for "Foundational Health" has never been greater.

This product is completely safe and effective. There is no contraindication with any medications. Seasilver may even help to offset some of the negative side effects of certain medications, such as chemotherapy and radiation. If your health care professional tells you its okay to eat food while taking your medication, then you can take this liquid nutritional supplement on a daily basis.

I didn't discover this product until I was well on my way to regaining my health. I researched several multiple vitamin and mineral supplements seeking one single product I could take on a daily basis that would provide the highest potency, quality and maximum absorption possible. Some were in capsule form and others in liquid or powder form. While these various products were quality supplements and I was confident were assisting me in building my immune system, I continued my research for even higher quality, properly balanced formulas, with proven immune enhancing ingredients. To date, this daily nutritional supplement surpasses all other capsule, powder or liquid nutritional supplements I have used over the last several years. It is a great tasting liquid that both adults and children will truly benefit from. My family consumes Seasilver and Sun Chlorella on a daily basis to achieve optimum nutrition.

Freeze-Dried Fruits and Vegetables

For those wishing to supplement their juicing program with quality freeze-dried fruits, vegetables and grains, please contact me. I will introduce you to a product backed by scientific research and study, and to a company that provides a product that surpasses unmitigated testing standards.

Exfoliating Gloves

The ultimate in bathing. We carry several different types, ranging from the basic nylon glove to the luxurious "sisal" body mit. Give your skin the clean it deserves each day! The gloves are economical, effective and last a very, very long time. In fact, the gloves become more abrasive and effective as they age.

Personal Care Products

After much research on the chemicals that are put into our personal care products, I realized that I was creating a toxic dump within my own body by using these products. When reading the labels on my personal care products I found at least two different chemicals that seemed to be common in most all products. These chemicals were Sodium Lauryl Sulfate and Propylene Glycol. Did you know in the industrial world Proplylene Glycol is used in antifreeze, brake and hydraulic fluid, airplane deicer, paint, floor wax, pet food, and tobacco? Sodium Lauryl Sulfate is used in engine degreasers, garage floor cleaners, car wash soaps as well as in "no more tears" baby shampoo! I couldn't believe that I used this to wash my baby's hair with as an infant. These findings triggered more research until I realized that the general American public doesn't truly understand the dangers of these chemicals as well as a host of others. Cancer has become an epidemic in the United States and chemicals play a huge factor behind the scenes, whether it is in the food we eat, the lotion we massage into our skin or the air we breathe. We are being bombarded with these toxins every day, all day.

After trying products from several companies, I located one company that is truly dedicated to the health of mankind. Shampoos, conditioners, toothpaste, cleansing gels, sunblock, and make-up, they have it all. It is a bit more expensive but well worth the cost. Cut corners in other areas of your life and purchase only safe personal care products. Check out our website for more details.

Samson Juicer

I have tried several types of juicers and find the Samson brand to be far superior to the others. This juicer is capable of not only juicing fruits and vegetables but also juicing wheatgrass as well as other grasses, an option not available on most juicers. It also serves as a meat and vegetable mincer and an oil extractor for your favorite seeds and nuts. The Samson juicer can also be used to make pasta, noodles, etc., from steamed rice.

This product is also equipped with a low-speed mill-type screw that preserves as much flavor and nutrition as possible. Other high-speed juicers destroy natural flavor and nutritional value.

If you are going to invest in your health, invest in a quality juicer that has multiple functions and that will provide you with the highest nutrition possible from your organic produce.

~

Medical Disclaimer

The information contained in this book is intended to provide helpful health information for those seeking a natural approach to treating chronic illness. It is made available with the understanding that the author and publisher are not engaged in rendering medical or psychological advice. The information should not be considered complete and should be used as a guideline in researching healthier alternatives in the treatment of disease on an individual basis. It should not be used in place of a call or visit to a medical, health or other competent professional

~

"A man's mind stretched by a new idea, can never go back to its original dimensions."
-Oliver Wendell Holmes

Your Thoughts

RESOURCE GUIDE

Physicians & Services

Chester V. Clark Jr., D.D.S.,M.P.H
Amity Dental Office
439 East Thompson
Amity, Arkansas   71921
Phone: 870-342-5265
Email: drcvcjr@alltel.net

   Service: › Dentist – Removal of Amalgam fillings

Kalpana D. Patel, M.D.,
F.A.A.P., F.A.A.E.M
Board Certified
65 Wehrle Drive
Buffalo, New York   14225
Phone: 716-833-2213
Fax: 716-833-2244

   Services: › Environmental Allergy &
               Occupational Medicine
             › Pure Nutritional Supplements

James Russell, D.C.
Chiropractor
6108 County Road 32
Norwich, New York 13815
Phone: 607-336-3434

Richard J. Ucci, M.D.
521 Main Street
P.O. Box 606
Oneonta, New York 13820
Phone: 607-432-8752

C. Samuel West, D.N., N.D.
Chemist and Lymphologist
P.O. Box 970266
Orem, Utah   84097
Phone: 800-975-0123

> Services: › Lymphology Certification Course
> › Author: *The Golden Seven Plus One*

Other Resources & Services

American Apiary Society
P.O. Box 54
Hartland Four Corners, Vermont 05249
Phone: 800-823-3460
Fax: 802-436-2827
International: 802-436-2708

> Service: › Venom Therapy Source

The Benton Sisters' Ministry
P.O. Box 552
Lakeport, California 95453
Phone: 707-262-0901
Fax: 707-263-5871
Email: team@bentonsisters.com
Web: www.bentonsisters.com

        Services: › Health Lectures
                         › Cooking Seminars
                         › Concerts

Tina Finneyfrock, Master Herbalist
5504 South Lebanon Rd.
Earlville, New York   13332
Phone: 315-691-3311
Email: tinfin@juno.com

        Services: › Apprentice Program
                         › Consultations
                         › Lectures
                         › Classes

Chemical Injury Information Network
P.O. Box 301
White Sulphur Springs, Montana 59645
Phone: 406-547-2255
Fax: 406-547-2455

National CFIDS Foundation
(Chronic Fatigue Immune Deficiency Syndrome)
103 Aletha Road
Needham, MA   02492
Phone: 781-449-3535
Fax: 781-449-8606
Web: www.ncf-net.org

Companies & Products (not listed on **Marpe′ Solutions** website)

Eagle Distributing Co.
7635 Main Street
Fishers, New York 14453
Phone: 800-825-5880
Phone: 716-924-2150
Fax: 716-924-0715
Web: www.homefiresafety.com
Email: info@homefiresafety.com

> Products: › The Phoenix System 2100
> › Fire Protection Systems

Heavenly Heat Saunas
1106 2nd Street
Encinitas, California 92024-5008
Phone: 800-697-2862
Email: heavenlyheat@home.com
Web: heavenlyheatsaunas.com

> Products: › Environmentally Safe Saunas

NEEDS   ‹ Call for Catalog ›
Nutritional, Ecological and
Environmental Delivery System
P.O. Box 580
East Syracuse, New York   13057
Phone: 800-634-1380
Fax: 800-295-NEED
Email: needs@needs.com
Web: www.needs.com

       Products: › Cello bags; Nutritional
                    Supplements; Personal Care
                    Products; Simple Soap; and
                    Air Cleaners

                         ~

*"Even if I should not follow the straight road
because of its straightness, I would follow it
because I have found by experience that when
all is said and done it is generally the happiest
and the most useful.*
                    -Michel Eyquem De Montaigne

Your Thoughts

BIBLIOGRAPHY

This suggested reading and resource list is provided for those wishing to explore an individual topic further. These are only a sampling of the many books I referenced throughout my healing process and writing this book. Some books may be out of print.

Appleton. *Lick The Sugar Habit*. Avery Publishing: 1989.

Astor, Stephen. *Hidden Food Allergies*. Avery Publishing: 1989.

Balch, James F. and Phyllis A. *Prescription For Nutritional*

　　Healing. Avery Publishing: 1990.

Blauer, Stephen. *The Juicing Book*. Avery Publishing: 1989.

Brecher, Harold and Arline. *Forty Something Forever, Guide To*

　　Chelation Therapy. Health Savers Press: 1992.

Buist, Robert. *Food Chemical Sensitivity*. Avery Publishing: 1988.

Carper, Jean. *Food-Your Miracle Medicine*. Harper-Collins: 1993.

Clark, Hulda Regehr, Dr. *The Cure For All Diseases*. New Century

　　Press: 1995.

Crook, William G., Dr. *The Yeast Connection Handbook.*

Professional Books: 1996.

- - -. *The Yeast Connection - A Medical Breakthrough.*

Vintage Books: 1986.

Dadd, Debra Lynn. *Nontoxic, Natural And Earthwise.*

Jeremy Tarcher: 1990.

Gioannini, Marilyn. *The Complete Food Allergy Cookbook.*

Prima Publishing: 1997.

Golan, Ralph Dr. *Optimal Wellness.* Ballantine Books,

Div. of Random House: 1995.

Golos, Natalie and Rea, William J., Dr. *Success In The Bedroom.*

Pinnacle Publishers: 1992.

Haas, Elson, M., Dr. *The Detox Diet.* Celestial Arts Publishing:

1996.

Heinerman, John. *Fruits And Vegetables.* Parker Publishing: 1995.

Hendricks, Greg. *Conscious Breathing.* Bantam: 1995.

Howard, Mary Ann. *Blueprint For Health.* Zondervan Publishing

House: 1985.

Jensen, Bernard, Dr. *Foods That Heal.* Avery Publishing: 1988.

Klein, Allen. *The Healing Power Of Humor*. Jeremy Tarcher: 1989.

Larimore, Bertha B. *Sprouting For All Seasons*. Horizon Publishers: 1975.

Leach, Robert A. and Phillips, Reed B. *The Chiropractic Theories*. 3rd ed. Lippincott, Williams and Wilkins: 1994.

Lust, John. *The Herb Book*. Bantam Books: 1974.

Monte, Tom. *The Complete Guide To Natural Healing*. Berkley Publishing Group: 1997.

Morton, Walker. *The Chelation Way*. Avery Publishing: 1990.

Murray, Michael and Pizzorno, Joseph. *Encyclopedia Of Natural Medicine*. Prima Publishing: 1998.

Null, Gary. *Utimate Anti-Aging Program*. Kensington Publishing: 1999.

Ott, John N. *Light, Radiation And You - How To Stay Healthy*. Devin-Adair Publishing: 1982.

Panos, M.B. and Heimlich, Jane. *Homeopathy At Home*. Jeremy Tarcher: 1980.

Passwater, Richard A. *Supernutrition*. Dial Press: 1985.

Rogers, Sherry, Dr. *The E.I. Syndrome*. Prestige Publishers: 1986.

Trowbridge, John Parks, Dr. and Walker, Morton. *The Yeast Syndrome*. Bantam Books: 1974.

Ullman, Dana. *Discover Homeopathy*. North Atlantic Books: 1991.

Weil, Andrew, Dr. *8 Weeks To Optimum Health*. Alfred A. Knopf: 1997.

West, C. Samuel, Dr. *The Golden Seven Plus One*. Samuel Publishing: 1981.

Wigmore, Ann. *The Wheatgrass Book*. Avery Publishing: 1985.

- - -. *Be Your Own Doctor*. Avery Publishing: 1983.

- - -. *Recipes For Longer Life*. Avery Publishing: 1982.

Wlodga, Ronad R. *Health Secrets From The Bible*. Triumph: 1979.

Zampieron, Eugene R., Dr. and Kamhi, Ellen. *The Natural Medicine Chest*. M. Evans and Company: 1999.

Ziff, Sam. *Silver Dental Fillings - The Toxic Timebomb*. Aurora Press: 1984.

ORDER INFORMATION

QUANTITY SALES

ATTENTION: Businesses, Organizations, Healing Centers, and Schools of Spiritual Development and Healthy Lifestyles

***Dying In The Land Of Plenty* is available at special quantity discounts** on bulk purchases for educational purposes or fund raising. Special books or book excerpts can also be created to fit specific needs.

Lectures, seminars, and one-on-one consultations are also available to large groups, small groups, and on an individual basis.

For all orders and information please contact:

Brenda O. Brown
Marpe´ Solutions
523 Granville Hill Road
Sherburne, New York 13460

Phone: (607) 674-9729
E-mail: marpesolutions@ascent.net
Website: www.marpesolutions.com

INDIVIDUAL SALES

Great Gift Idea! If you have read this book and find it interesting and helpful, pass it on to a friend. Better yet, purchase additional copies and give the "gift of hope and renewed health" to your friends and loved ones. (For your convenience, an Order Form is provided on the next page.)

ORDER TODAY!

ORDER FORM

(Original price $19.95 —use this Order Form and save $2.00 per book)

☐ **YES!** Please send me _____ copy(ies) of

DYING IN THE LAND OF PLENTY
UNVEILING THE SHROUD OF DISEASE

At $17.95 each $ _____
Plus $4.50 shipping & handling per book $ _____
NY State residents, add 7% sales tax $ _____
                              Total: $ _____

Please make   ☐ Check or ☐ Money Order payable to:

MARPE´ SOLUTIONS

Name _____

Address _____

City _____ **State** _____ **Zip Code** _____

Phone: _____ **E-mail:** _____

Please send Order Form with Payment to:

Brenda O. Brown
Marpe´ Solutions
523 Granville Road
Sherburne, New York   13460

(Please allow 2-4 weeks for delivery)

THANK YOU FOR YOUR ORDER!